T0177499

50 Studies Every Ophthalmologist Should Know

50 STUDIES EVERY DOCTOR SHOULD KNOW

50 Studies Every Doctor Should Know: The Key Studies that Form the
Foundation of Evidence Based Medicine, Revised Edition
Michael E. Hochman

50 Studies Every Internist Should Know
*Kristopher Swiger, Joshua R. Thomas, Michael E. Hochman,
and Steven Hochman*

50 Studies Every Neurologist Should Know
David Y. Hwang and David M. Greer

50 Studies Every Pediatrician Should Know
*Ashaunta T. Anderson, Nina L. Shapiro, Stephen C. Aronoff,
Jeremiah Davis, and Michael Levy*

50 Imaging Studies Every Doctor Should Know
Christoph I. Lee

50 Studies Every Surgeon Should Know
SreyRam Kuy, Rachel J. Kwon, and Miguel A. Burch

50 Studies Every Intensivist Should Know
Edward A. Bittner

50 Studies Every Palliative Care Doctor Should Know
David Hui, Akhila Reddy, and Eduardo Bruera

50 Studies Every Psychiatrist Should Know
Ish P. Bhalla, Rajesh R. Tampi, and Vinod H. Srihari

50 Studies Every Anesthesiologist Should Know
Anita Gupta, Michael E. Hochman, and Elena N. Gutman

50 Studies Every Ophthalmologist Should Know
Alan D. Penman, Kimberly W. Crowder, and William M. Watkins, Jr.

50 Studies Every Ophthalmologist Should Know

ALAN D. PENMAN, MD, PHD, MPH
Department of Preventive Medicine, John D. Bower School of Population Health
Department of Ophthalmology, School of Medicine
University of Mississippi Medical Center
Jackson, MS

KIMBERLY W. CROWDER
Department of Ophthalmology, School of Medicine
University of Mississippi Medical Center
Jackson, MS

WILLIAM M. WATKINS, JR.
Department of Ophthalmology, School of Medicine
University of Mississippi Medical Center
Jackson, MS

SERIES EDITOR
MICHAEL E. HOCHMAN, MD, MPH
Associate Professor, Medicine
Director, Gehr Family Center for Health Systems Science
USC Keck School of Medicine
Los Angeles, CA

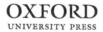

OXFORD
UNIVERSITY PRESS

OXFORD
UNIVERSITY PRESS

Oxford University Press is a department of the University of Oxford. It furthers
the University's objective of excellence in research, scholarship, and education
by publishing worldwide. Oxford is a registered trade mark of Oxford University
Press in the UK and certain other countries.

Published in the United States of America by Oxford University Press
198 Madison Avenue, New York, NY 10016, United States of America.

© Oxford University Press 2020

All rights reserved. No part of this publication may be reproduced, stored in
a retrieval system, or transmitted, in any form or by any means, without the
prior permission in writing of Oxford University Press, or as expressly permitted
by law, by license, or under terms agreed with the appropriate reproduction
rights organization. Inquiries concerning reproduction outside the scope of the
above should be sent to the Rights Department, Oxford University Press, at the
address above.

You must not circulate this work in any other form
and you must impose this same condition on any acquirer.

Library of Congress Cataloging-in-Publication Data
Names: Penman, Alan D., author. | Crowder, Kimberly W., author. |
Watkins, William M., Jr. (William Marvin), 1981– author.
Title: 50 studies every ophthalmologist should know / Alan D. Penman,
Kimberly W. Crowder, William M. Watkins, Jr.
Other titles: Fifty studies every ophthalmologist should know |
50 studies every doctor should know (Series)
Description: New York, NY : Oxford University Press, [2020] |
Series: Fifty studies every doctor should know |
Includes bibliographical references and index.
Identifiers: LCCN 2019053607 (print) | LCCN 2019053608 (ebook) |
ISBN 9780190050726 (paperback) | ISBN 9780190050740 (epub)
Subjects: MESH: Eye Diseases | Evidence-Based Medicine |
Clinical Trials as Topic | Case Reports
Classification: LCC RE46 (print) | LCC RE46 (ebook) |
NLM WW 140 | DDC 617.7—dc23
LC record available at https://lccn.loc.gov/2019053607
LC ebook record available at https://lccn.loc.gov/2019053608

This material is not intended to be, and should not be considered, a substitute for medical or other
professional advice. Treatment for the conditions described in this material is highly dependent on the
individual circumstances. And, while this material is designed to offer accurate information with respect to the
subject matter covered and to be current as of the time it was written, research and knowledge about medical
and health issues is constantly evolving and dose schedules for medications are being revised continually, with
new side effects recognized and accounted for regularly. Readers must therefore always check the product
information and clinical procedures with the most up-to-date published product information and data sheets
provided by the manufacturers and the most recent codes of conduct and safety regulation. The publisher
and the authors make no representations or warranties to readers, express or implied, as to the accuracy
or completeness of this material. Without limiting the foregoing, the publisher and the authors make no
representations or warranties as to the accuracy or efficacy of the drug dosages mentioned in the material.
The authors and the publisher do not accept, and expressly disclaim, any responsibility for any liability, loss,
or risk that may be claimed or incurred as a consequence of the use and/or application of any of the contents
of this material.

9 8 7 6 5 4 3 2 1

Printed by Marquis, Canada

CONTENTS

PREFACE

In the last 40 years ophthalmology has become an increasingly important field of medicine. When we first became aware of the "50 Studies" series, it was obvious that there was a need for a concise summary of the ophthalmology literature that every ophthalmologist should know. Selecting which studies to include was, of course, a challenge; rather than studies that are most frequently cited, we decided to focus on landmark studies that changed thinking and practice in the field. Most are prospective, randomized controlled trials that have helped shape current ophthalmology practice guidelines; wherever possible, we have included a reference to the practice guidelines of the American Academy of Ophthalmology. However, some important observational (cohort, case-control, and descriptive) studies are also included. To the authors' knowledge, there is no other book on the market that succinctly summarizes the clinically relevant ophthalmology literature that every ophthalmologist should be familiar with. The book should be a useful source for ophthalmologists in training or preparing for board review, a quick reference for practitioners, and helpful for those studying the historical development of ophthalmology practice.

The book is not aimed solely at ophthalmologists, however. Every practicing physician, no matter his or her specialty, should be familiar with the relation of the eye to the rest of the human body, and with the use and value of the ophthalmoscope. To paraphrase a well-known saying, the eyes are a window to the brain and the vascular system. Ophthalmology has a particular relevance to physicians working in primary care, internal medicine, neurology, neurosurgery, pediatrics, and emergency medicine.

We thought that it might be a useful learning exercise for our ophthalmology residents to be involved in the search for relevant papers and the writing of drafts, and they agreed. We thank them for their hard work and contributions: Sneh Dhannawat (PGY-2, 2018), Jonathan Feng (PGY-2, 2018), Lee Jones (PGY-2, 2018), Jeffrey St. John (PGY-2, 2018), Jack Bullock (PGY-3, 2018), Jonathan Carrere (PGY-3, 2018), Jorge Jimenez (PGY-3, 2018), David Kilpatrick (PGY-4, 2018), Ben Pace (PGY-4, 2018), Devin Tran (PGY-4, 2018), Sean Carter (PGY-2, 2019), Kevin Mays (PGY-2, 2019), Clayton Patrick (PGY-2, 2019), and Erin Petersen (PGY-2, 2019). We hope they learned some valuable lessons about writing and editing!

Alan D. Penman
Kimberly W. Crowder
William M. Watkins, Jr.

1

Effectiveness of Histocompatibility Matching in High-Risk Corneal Transplantation[*]

Collaborative Cornea Transplant Studies (CCTS)

These studies demonstrate that, for high-risk patients who are immunosuppressed by topical steroid therapy and followed up according to
CCTS protocol: (1) neither HLA-A, -B, nor HLA-DR antigen matching
substantially reduced the likelihood of corneal graft failure; (2) a positive donor-recipient crossmatch does not dramatically increase the risk
of corneal graft failure; and (3) ABO blood group matching, which can
be achieved with relatively little effort and expense, may be effective in
reducing the risk of graft failure.

—STARK ET AL[1]

Research Question: Does matching HLA-A, -B, and/or HLA-DR antigens,
donor-recipient crossmatching, or ABO compatibility reduce the risk of corneal
allograft rejection and failure in high-risk patients?[1]

Funding: National Eye Institute, National Institutes of Health.

Year Study Began: 1986.

Year Study Published: 1992.

[*]Basic and Clinical Science Course, Section 8. *External Disease and Cornea*. San Francisco: American
Academy of Ophthalmology; 2018–2019.

Study Location: 6 centers in the United States.

Who Was Studied: Patients, at least 10 years of age, needing a corneal graft, with uncompromised immune systems and at high risk for corneal graft rejection. The cornea was required to have two or more quadrants of corneal stromal vascularization and/or a history of prior corneal graft rejection.

Who Was Excluded: Patients who had systemic immunologic disorders, were on immunosuppressive medications, needed immediate corneal transplantation, or had conditions likely to cause nonrejection graft failure were excluded.

How Many Patients: 419 in the Antigen Matching Study (AMS) and 32 in the Crossmatch Study (CS).

Study Overview: The Collaborative Cornea Transplant Studies (CCTS) consisted of two trials, the AMS and the CS (Figure 1.1).[1,2]

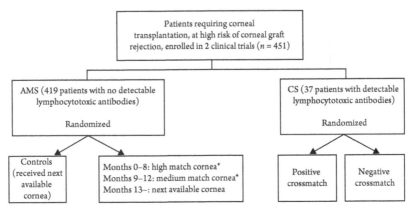

Figure 1.1 Summary of the CCTS.
*High match: corneas from donors matching three or four HLA-A, -B antigens or two HLA-DR antigens; medium match: corneas from donors matching two or more HLA-A, -B antigens.

    The AMS was a prospective, double-masked, clinical trial of patients with no detectable lymphocytotoxic antibodies grafted with varying degrees of HLA-matched corneas. (If a patient's serum was cytotoxic to 20% of cells, then it was considered to have detectable lymphocytotoxic antibodies.) The aim was to assess the effect of HLA-A, -B, and HLA-DR antigen matching on corneal graft survival. The CS was a prospective, randomized, double-masked, clinical trial of patients with detectable lymphocytotoxic antibodies given corneal grafts from positively or negatively crossmatched donors. (A positive crossmatch indicated that the recipient had cytotoxic antibodies toward the donor cornea.) The aim was to assess the effect of crossmatching on corneal graft survival.

Study Intervention: In the AMS, all patients received corneas from negatively cross-matched donors, and without regard for ABO type. Ninety percent of patients (the treatment group) were eligible to receive corneas from donors with 3 or 4 antigens matching HLA-A and HLA-B or two antigens from HLA-DR class (high match). Any patient not allocated a cornea by 8 months became eligible for corneas from donors matching only 2 or more HLA-A, -B antigens (low match). If no cornea had been allocated by 12 months, the patient was assigned the next available cornea. Ten percent served as controls and randomly received the next available cornea through the United Network for Organ Sharing.

In the CS, patients were randomly assigned to the positive or negative crossmatch group when they first demonstrated a positive crossmatch against a cornea donor. If randomized to the positive group, the patient received one of the current donor's two corneas; the second cornea went to a patient who had a negative crossmatch with the current donor and who had previously been randomly assigned to the negative group. If randomized to the negative group, the patient waited for a cornea procured at a later date.

All patients were treated with topical steroids after surgery. The dosage of prednisolone acetate, 1.0%, was reduced from every 2 hours while awake for the first 3 postoperative days to 6 times daily on the 4th day, to 4 times daily on the 15th day, to three times daily at 2 months, to twice daily at 3 months, and to once daily at 4 months. Dexamethasone ointment was used at bedtime for the first month. Treatment with fluorometholone, 0.1%, was tapered from 4 times daily at 5 months to twice daily at 6 months, to once daily at 7 months and thereafter.

Follow-Up: 5 years (maximum).

Endpoints: The primary outcome for both the AMS and CS was the time to irreversible corneal graft failure secondary to any cause. Secondary outcomes were time to first immunologic graft reaction, time to graft failure secondary to allograft rejection, and visual acuity.

RESULTS

Antigen Matching Study

- The incidence of graft failure was similar in the HLA-A and HLA-B high and low match groups ($P = .35$). At 3 years after surgery, 37% of the grafts

in the low match group and 33% of the grafts in the high match group had
failed.
- The low and high match groups had similar rates of graft reaction
  ($P = .38$). By 3 years after surgery, 66% of the low match group and 64% of
  the high match group had had a graft reaction.
  - By 3 years after surgery, 26% of low match and 21% of high match grafts
    had failed due to graft rejection ($P = .34$).
- The HLA-DR high and low match groups had nearly identical rates of graft
  failure ($P = .95$).
  - The proportion of eyes having at least one graft reaction was also similar
    between the HLA-DR comparison groups ($P = .77$).
- At 3 years after surgery, 24% of the grafts in the low match group and 25%
  of the grafts in the high match group had failed due to rejection ($P = .60$).
- The ABO-incompatible group had slightly more graft failures than the
  ABO-compatible group ($P = .27$).
  - At 3 years after surgery, 41% of the grafts in the incompatible group and
    34% of the grafts in the compatible group had failed.
- The ABO-incompatible group had a slightly larger proportion of patients
  with graft reaction ($P = .24$).
  - At 3 years after surgery, 68% of the incompatible group and 64% of the
    compatible group had had at least one reaction.
  - At 3 years after surgery, 30% of the incompatible group and 22% of the
    compatible group had graft failures due to rejection.

Crossmatch Study

- The positive and negative groups had a similar incidence of graft failures
  ($P = .66$).
  - At 2 years after surgery, 36% of grafts in the positive group and 45% in
    the negative group had failed.
- The positive and negative groups had similar rates of graft reaction
  ($P = .83$).
  - At 2 years after surgery, 55% of the positive group and 61% of the
    negative group had had a graft reaction.
  - The rate of graft failure due to rejection was much higher in the negative
    group than in the positive group ($P = .33$). At 2 years after surgery, 16%
    of grafts in the positive group and 38% in the negative group had failed
    due to rejection.

Criticism and Limitations: The postoperative topical immunosuppressive regimen used in the CCTS was more intensive than that used in other recent studies
showing an effect of HLA matching on corneal graft survival. A beneficial effect
of HLA matching on graft survival may have been abrogated in the CCTS by
postoperative steroid therapy.[3]

The number of patients in the CS study was small ($n = 37$). Furthermore, the
racial/ethnic composition of the donor and patient groups in both the AMS and
CS was more diverse than that reported for many of the other studies, and this
made accurate histocompatibility assignment and matching difficult. HLA-DQ
alleles, which may also be important with regard to donor rejection, were not
studied. Minor histocompatibility antigens, which have been demonstrated to
play a role in graft rejection in mice, were not studied.

Two additional factors that may have contributed to the relatively high success rate for penetrating keratoplasty in the CCTS were a vigorous educational
program to assure medication compliance, and frequent, regular follow-up
examinations by the transplanting surgeon.[3]

Other Relevant Studies and Information:

- The benefit of HLA matching in corneal transplantation remains
  a subject of debate. The authors of a 2015 review state: "There
  is [sic] enough data to show that when proper DNA-based
  typing techniques are being used, even low-risk perforating
  corneal transplantations benefit from matching for HLA Class I,
  and high-risk cases from HLA Class I and probably Class II
  matching. Combining HLA class I and class II matching, or using
  the HLAMatchmaker could further improve the effect of HLA
  matching."[4]
- In a recent randomized, double-blind clinical trial comparing HLA
  matching and random graft assignment in 639 normal-risk and high-risk
  patients, HLA matching did not show a significant advantage.[5]
  - The estimated cumulative incidence rate of immune reactions
    after 2 years was 15.7% in the HLA matching arm and 17% in the
    control arm.

Summary and Implications: These studies demonstrated that, for high-risk
patients who are immunosuppressed by topical steroid therapy: (1) neither

HLA-A, HLA-B, nor HLA-DR antigen matching substantially reduced the likelihood of corneal graft failure; (2) a positive donor-recipient crossmatch did not increase the risk of corneal graft failure; and (3) ABO blood group matching may be effective in reducing the risk of graft failure from rejection. Intensive steroid therapy after transplantation, frequent follow-up, medication and follow-up compliance, and patient education appear to play a significant role in corneal graft success. Further analysis and standardization is needed regarding postoperative steroid treatment and the role of microhistocompatibility antigens and other major histocompatibility complex (MHC) antigens.

CLINICAL CASE: A YOUNG MAN NEEDING A REPEAT CORNEAL GRAFT

Case History

A 38-year-old African American man presents to you for a repeat corneal transplant evaluation. He experienced eye trauma 5 years ago, requiring a penetrating keratoplasty, and the current graft has subsequently failed. He has no other medical issues and is without known immune compromise. How would you counsel the tissue bank in regard to donor selection?

A. No regard for HLA or ABO compatibility is needed.
B. Request that the donor cornea be closely matched for HLA compatibility alone.
C. Request that the donor cornea be closely matched for ABO compatibility alone.
D. Request that the donor cornea be closely matched for both HLA and ABO compatibility.

Suggested Answer

Option C.

ABO compatibility may decrease rejection in high-risk immunocompetent patients. For high-risk patients who are immunosuppressed by topical steroid therapy and followed up according to CCTS protocol, studies show that: (1) neither HLA-A, HLA-B, nor HLA-DR antigen matching substantially reduces the likelihood of corneal graft failure; (2) a positive donor-recipient crossmatch does not dramatically increase the risk of corneal graft failure; and (3) ABO blood group matching, which can be achieved with relatively little effort and expense, may be effective in reducing the risk of graft failure.

References

1. The collaborative corneal transplantation studies (CCTS). Effectiveness of histocompatibility matching in high-risk corneal transplantation. The Collaborative Corneal Transplantation Studies Research Group. *Arch Ophthalmol.* 1992;110(10):1392–403.
2. Design and methods of the collaborative corneal transplantation studies. The Collaborative Corneal Transplantation Studies Research Group. *Cornea.* 1993;12(2):93–103.
3. Sugar J. The Collaborative Corneal Transplantation Studies. *Arch Ophthalmol.* 1992;110(11):1517–8.
4. van Essen TH, Roelen DL, Williams KA, Jager MJ. Matching for human leukocyte antigens (HLA) in corneal transplantation—to do or not to do. *Prog Retin Eye Res.* 2015;46:84–110.
5. Böhringer D, Grotejohann B, Ihorst G, Reinshagen H, Spierings E, Reinhard T. Rejection prophylaxis in corneal transplant. *Dtsch Arztebl Int.* 2018;115(15):259–65.

2

Topical Corticosteroids for Herpes Simplex Stromal Keratitis*

The Herpetic Eye Disease Study (HEDS)

The topical corticosteroid regimen used in this study was significantly better than placebo in reducing persistence or progression of stromal inflammation and in shortening the duration of herpes simplex stromal keratitis.

—Wilhelmus et al[1]

Research Question: How effective are topical corticosteroids as adjunctive therapy in the treatment of herpes simplex stromal keratitis?[1]

Funding: National Eye Institute, National Institutes of Health.

Year Study Began: 1989.

Year Study Published: 1994.

Study Location: 9 clinical centers in the United States.

Who Was Studied: Patients 12 years of age or older with active stromal keratitis consistent with herpes simplex virus (HSV) (defined as an area of at least

---

* Basic and Clinical Science Course, Section 8. *External Disease and Cornea*. San Francisco: American Academy of Ophthalmology; 2018–2019: 216, 222–223.

2.5 mm² of active corneal stromal inflammation with diffuse or disciform inflammatory stromal edema [non-necrotizing] or a dense, opaque, inflammatory infiltration [necrotizing]), who had not received any topical or systemic corticosteroids within the prior 10 days.

Who Was Excluded: Patients were excluded if there was active HSV epithelial keratitis or an epithelial defect larger than 1.0 mm in the involved eye; prior corneal transplant in the involved eye; or prior adverse reaction to prednisolone phosphate or trifluridine. Patients who developed trifluridine toxicity at week 7 and were switched to a different antiviral were excluded, as were those who suffered an adverse event, including development of a dendritic epithelial keratitis after starting the topical antiviral, follicular conjunctivitis, allergic conjunctivitis, or development of an epithelial defect.

How Many Patients: 106.

Study Overview: The Herpetic Eye Disease Study (HEDS I; HEDS-SKN) was a randomized, double-masked, placebo-controlled clinical trial (Figure 2.1).[1,2]

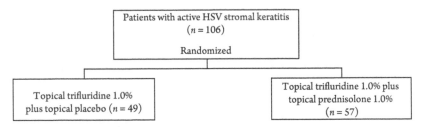

Figure 2.1. Summary of HEDS.

Study Intervention: Patients were assigned to either topical prednisolone phosphate or placebo. Both groups received topical trifluridine 1% 4 times daily for 3 weeks then twice daily for 7 weeks. Patients assigned to the steroid group received, in addition, topical prednisolone 1% 8 times daily in the first week, with tapering over the next 9 weeks. Patients assigned to the placebo group followed an identical dosing schedule.

Follow-Up: 6 months.

Endpoints: The primary endpoints were time to treatment failure, defined by specific criteria as persistent or progressive stromal keratitis/uveitis or an adverse event (dendritic epithelial keratitis, allergic or follicular conjunctivitis, corneal epithelial erosions or defect), and time to treatment success, defined as resolution of stromal keratitis/uveitis. Secondary endpoints were visual acuity and recurrence of HSV eye disease (dendritic epithelial keratitis during study treatment or any form of herpes simplex eye disease after discontinuation of treatment).

RESULTS

- Compared with placebo, corticosteroid therapy reduced the risk of persistent or progressive stromal keratouveitis by 68%.
  - Fifteen patients (26%) in the steroid group and 36 patients (73%) in the placebo group were treatment failures before completing the 10-week course of trial medications.
  - By 16 weeks, 28 patients (49%) in the steroid group and 37 patients (76%) in the placebo group had failed treatment.
  - The median time to treatment failure was 98 days for the steroid group and 17 days for the placebo group ($P < 0.001$).
- When all patients were considered, including those whose keratitis resolved with trial medications and those removed from the trial and treated at the ophthalmologist's discretion, the time from randomization to resolution of active herpes simplex keratitis was significantly shorter overall for the steroid group (26 days) than the placebo group (72 days) ($P < 0.001$).
- At 6 months, no clinically or statistically significant differences in visual outcome were identified between the steroid and placebo groups.
  - 59% of eyes in the placebo group and 61% of eyes in the steroid group had an improvement in visual acuity of 2 lines or more on the Bailey-Lovie chart.
  - 67% of each group had a best-corrected visual acuity of 20/40 or better at 6 months.
- At 6 months, there was no significant difference in the frequency of recurrent stromal keratitis between the steroid and placebo groups ($P = 0.9$).

Criticisms and Limitations: The researchers used a clinical rather than a virologic case definition. However, the percentage of patients reporting a history of previous herpes simplex eye or nasolabial disease was approximately similar in the two treatment groups, and this limitation is unlikely to have biased the results significantly.

The 10-week tapered regimen of corticosteroids may be too brief for many patients. The authors suggest that therapy may need to be tapered more slowly for most patients with herpes simplex stromal keratitis.

Other Relevant Studies and Information:

- A previous placebo-controlled clinical trial of 30 patients showed similar results in that long-term visual acuity was unaffected, but topical corticosteroids (at a fixed dose) hastened resolution of herpes simplex disciform stromal keratitis.[3]
- The HEDS II study (HEDS-SKS), a randomized, double-masked, placebo-controlled trial in 104 patients with HSV stromal keratitis without epithelial keratitis, showed that oral acyclovir in addition to topical corticosteroids and trifluridine was of no additional benefit, but the group receiving oral acyclovir did show improvement in visual acuity at 6 months compared to placebo.[4]
- The HEDS III study (HEDS-IRT), a randomized clinical trial to evaluate the addition of oral acyclovir to a regimen of topical prednisolone phosphate and trifluridine for the treatment of iridocyclitis, showed a trend in the results suggestive of a benefit of oral acyclovir.[5]
  - A treatment failure occurred in 11 (50%) of the 22 patients in the acyclovir-treated group and in 19 (68%) of the 28 patients in the placebo group.
- A subsequent HEDS study to evaluate the efficacy of a 3-week course of oral acyclovir in *preventing* stromal keratitis or iritis in patients with HSV epithelial keratitis showed no apparent benefit in preventing HSV stromal keratitis or iritis during the subsequent year.[6]

Summary and Implications: Topical corticosteroids can be used judiciously with protective antiviral cover in the acute treatment of patients with herpes simplex stromal keratitis who have not recently received corticosteroid therapy to reduce persistence or progression of stromal inflammation and shorten the duration of herpes simplex stromal keratitis. However, topical corticosteroid use can be postponed in some patients during careful observation for a few weeks; this may delay resolution of stromal keratitis but has no detrimental effect on visual acuity at 6 months.

CLINICAL CASE: A MIDDLE-AGED MAN WITH HERPES SIMPLEX STROMAL KERATITIS

Case History

A 48-year-old white man presents to your clinic complaining of blurring of vision and severe pain in the left eye. He denies any trauma, but feels as if there is some dirt under his eyelid. He is mildly sensitive to light. He denies any contact lens use or recent bathing in lakes or hot tubs. He states that this has happened to him in the past, and he was told it was due to herpes. He took antiviral medicines at that time which led to its resolution. He has no complaints about the fellow eye.

On examination, all findings are normal in his right eye. His left eye visual acuity is 20/100 with an intraocular pressure (IOP) of 22 mm Hg. Pupil exam, confrontation visual field, and extraocular movements are normal. Anterior slit lamp exam reveals a dense, opaque, paracentral infiltrate of approximately 1 × 3 mm with surrounding edema. There is an associated 0.5 mm epithelial defect overlying the infiltrate. No pigmentation or satellite lesions are noted. Dilated fundus exam is normal. Corneal scraping is performed and sent for gram stain and culture. The gram stain returns negative.

After initiating acyclovir 400 mg x5 daily PO, the patient returns to your clinic with the foreign body sensation improving and resolution of his epithelial defect; however, his vision is unchanged. The culture shows no growth to date. What is the next step in management for the patient?

A. Continue present management.
B. Add a topical antibiotic.
C. Add fortified antibiotics.
D. Add a topical corticosteroid.

Suggested Answer

The findings suggest necrotizing herpes simplex stromal keratitis. Since he has shown a good response to the oral antiviral treatment, and the culture is not indicative of a bacterial etiology, a topical corticosteroid (option D) may hasten the recovery of his cornea.

References

1. Wilhelmus KR, Gee L, Hauck WW, et al. Herpetic Eye Disease Study: a controlled trial of topical corticosteroids for herpes simplex stromal keratitis. *Ophthalmology.* 1994;101(12):1883–95; discussion 1895–6.
2. Dawson CR, Jones DB, Kaufman HE, Barron BA, Hauck WW, Wilhelmus KR. Design and organization of the herpetic eye disease study (HEDS). *Curr Eye Res.* 1991;10 Suppl:105–10.
3. Power WJ, Hillary MP, Benedict-Smith A, Collum LM. Acyclovir ointment plus topical betamethasone or placebo in first episode disciform keratitis. *Br J Ophthalmol.* 1992;76: 711–13.
4. Barron BA, Gee L, Hauck WW, et al. Herpetic Eye Disease Study: a controlled trial of oral acyclovir for herpes simplex stromal keratitis. *Ophthalmology.* 1994;101(12):1871–82.
5. A controlled trial of oral acyclovir for iridocyclitis caused by herpes simplex virus. The Herpetic Eye Disease Study Group. *Arch Ophthalmol.* 1996;114(9):1065–72.
6. A controlled trial of oral acyclovir for the prevention of stromal keratitis or iritis in patients with herpes simplex virus epithelial keratitis. The Epithelial Keratitis Trial. The Herpetic Eye Disease Study Group. *Arch Ophthalmol.* 1997;115(6):703–12. Erratum in *Arch Ophthalmol.* 1997;115(9):1196.

Topical Corticosteroids for Bacterial Keratitis*

The Steroids for Corneal Ulcers Trial (SCUT)

> Adjunctive topical corticosteroid use does not improve 3-month vision
> in patients with bacterial corneal ulcers.
>
> —SRINIVASAN ET AL[1]

Research Question: Are topical corticosteroids beneficial as an adjunctive therapy when treating bacterial corneal ulcers with topical antibiotics?[1]

Funding: National Eye Institute, National Institutes of Health.

Year Study Began: 2006.

Year Study Published: 2012.

Study Location: 5 centers in the United States and India.

Who Was Studied: Patients with a culture-positive bacterial corneal ulcer treated for at least 48 hours with topical moxifloxacin 0.5%.

Who Was Excluded: Patients were excluded if there was a corneal perforation or impending perforation, evidence of fungal or *Acanthamoeba* infection, evidence of herpes keratitis by history or exam, use of a topical corticosteroid or systemic

* Basic and Clinical Science Course, Section 8. *External Disease and Cornea.* San Francisco: American Academy of Ophthalmology; 2018–2019: 272.

prednisolone during the course of the present ulcer, previous penetrating keratoplasty, previous corneal scar in the affected eye, or vision less than 20/200 in
the fellow eye.

How Many Patients: 500.

Study Overview: The Steroids for Corneal Ulcers Trial (SCUT) was a randomized, placebo-controlled, double masked clinical trial (Figure 3.1).[1,2]

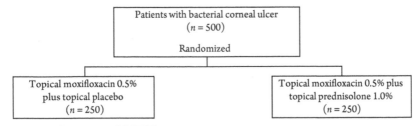

Figure 3.1. Summary of SCUT.

Study Intervention: Patients were randomly allocated to receive topical prednisolone or placebo. The corticosteroid group was given topical prednisolone sodium phosphate 1.0% one drop 4 times daily for 1 week, 2 times daily for 1 week,
and then once daily for 1 week; the placebo regimen was identical. The regimen
for moxifloxacin in both groups consisted of one drop each hour while awake for
the first 48 hours, then every 2 hours until reepithelialization, then 4 times daily
until 3 weeks from enrollment.

Follow-Up: 3 months.

Endpoints: The primary measure of outcome was best spectacle-corrected
visual acuity (BSCVA) at 3 months from enrollment using a tumbling E chart.
Secondary outcomes included BSCVA at 3 weeks, infiltrate/scar size at 3 weeks
and 3 months by slit lamp exam, time to reepithelialization, and rate of adverse
events including corneal perforation, rise in intraocular pressure (IOP).

RESULTS

- At 3 months, corticosteroids offered no significant improvement in
  BSCVA compared with placebo, controlling for baseline BSCVA ($P = .82$).

- At 3 weeks, corticosteroid-treated patients had .024 better logMAR acuity (approximately one-fourth of a line), controlling for baseline BSCVA ($P = .49$).
- Corticosteroid use was not associated with a statistically significant difference in infiltrate/scar size at either 3 weeks ($P = .60$) or 3 months ($P = .40$).
- Median time to reepithelialization was 7.0 days in the placebo arm and 7.5 days in the corticosteroid arm ($P = .25$).
  - After adjusting for baseline epithelial defect size, there was no significant difference in time to reepithelialization in the 2 arms in the first 21 days of the trial ($P = .44$).
  - Although more patients in the corticosteroid arm had an epithelial defect at 21 days or later compared with placebo (17.6% vs. 10.8%; $P = .04$), there was no difference in healing by 3 months between the treatment arms ($P = .73$).
- There was no significant difference between treatment arms in the number of corneal perforations ($P > .99$) or number of penetrating keratoplasties ($P > .99$).
- The use of corticosteroids was not associated with an increase in IOP.
  - Surprisingly, an increase in IOP between 25 and 35 mm Hg was observed more often in the placebo group (10 vs. 2 patients [$P = .04$]). IOP was never observed to be more than 35 mm Hg in either group.

Prespecified subgroup analyses

- In patients with baseline BSCVA of counting fingers or worse, corticosteroid-treated patients had .17 better logMAR acuity (approximately 1.7 lines) compared with placebo at 3 months ($P = .03$).
- In ulcers completely covering the central 4 mm pupil, corticosteroid-treated patients had .20 better logMAR acuity (approximately 2 lines) compared with placebo at 3 months ($P = .02$).
- In ulcers with the deepest infiltrates (> 67% depth) at baseline, corticosteroid-treated patients had .15 better logMAR acuity (approximately 1.5 lines) compared with placebo at 3 months ($P = .07$).

Criticisms and Limitations: More central corneal ulcers encompassing the entire 4-mm pupil were observed in the corticosteroid group than in the placebo group ($P = .02$). Ulcers that were completely covering the 4-mm pupil were larger than those partially covering it or existing entirely in the periphery; the former type yielded worse visual acuity. However, the analyses controlled for baseline visual acuity and baseline infiltrate/scar size, and it is unlikely that differences in the location of the ulcer at baseline significantly biased the results.

The treatment regimen was standardized and not as aggressive as it might have been; it is possible that an increased frequency or duration of corticosteroid use could have a larger effect. Also, a commonly used broad-spectrum fluoroquinolone was used, which may not have been the most efficacious choice for each patient. Physicians were allowed to change or add antibiotics at any time if they thought it was medically necessary. The rate of antibiotic change was approximately 15% in both arms of the trial, however.

Most ulcers in this trial occurred in individuals enrolled in India and not wearing contact lenses. Furthermore, the distribution of organisms was different between the United States and India: most *Nocardia* spp. were isolated from Indian patients. However, the two treatment arms were well balanced for most baseline characteristics, including the distribution of organisms, and the results of this trial can be generalized to other populations.

Other Relevant Studies and Information:

- In a follow-up study of SCUT, 399 of the original 500 patients were evaluated at 12 months.[3] Results showed that adjunctive topical corticosteroid therapy may be associated with improved long-term clinical outcomes in bacterial corneal ulcers not caused by *Nocardia* species.
  - In patients with non-*Nocardia* ulcers, corticosteroid use was associated with a mean 1-line improvement (−.10 logMAR) in BSCVA at 12 months ($P = .02$). No significant difference was observed in 12-month BSCVA for *Nocardia* ulcers (.18 logMAR, $P = .16$).
  - Corticosteroids were associated with larger mean scar size (.47 mm) at 12 months among *Nocardia* ulcers ($P = .02$); no significant difference was identified by treatment for scar size for non-*Nocardia* ulcers ($P = .46$).

Summary and Implications: In general, topical corticosteroids initiated within 3 days of presentation as adjunctive therapy after at least 48 hours of antibiotic usage in the treatment of non-*Nocardia* bacterial corneal ulcers do not show any short-term benefit but may be associated with improved long-term clinical outcomes. There is some evidence of short-term benefit in patients with baseline BSCVA of counting fingers or worse, with ulcers completely covering the central

4-mm pupil, and in ulcers with the infiltrates > 67% of the full corneal thickness at baseline. Further study is needed.

Note: These results should not be extrapolated to patients with other infectious etiologies of keratitis, such as fungus, herpes viruses, *Acanthamoeba*, or atypical mycobacteria, and these entities should be excluded before considering adjunctive steroid therapy.

CLINICAL CASE: A YOUNG MAN WITH A BACTERIAL CORNEAL ULCER

Case History
A 35-year-old man presents to your clinic complaining of blurring of vision, severe pain, and sensitivity to light in his right eye. He does not remember getting dust or grit in the eye, but feels like he has something in his eye. He does not wear contact lenses. He has a history of mild symptomatic dry eye disease controlled with artificial tears, but no other history of eye disease or eye surgeries. He denies any recent swimming in lakes or hot tubs. He has no complaints for the fellow eye.

On examination, all findings are normal in his left eye. His right eye visual acuity is 20/200 with an IOP of 22 mm Hg. Pupil exam, confrontation visual field, and extraocular movements are normal. Anterior slit lamp exam reveals a small (3 mm), circular, central, white infiltrate of the anterior corneal stroma with slight thinning and an overlying epithelial defect. There is no pigmentation or feather-like appearance to the opacity. Dilated fundus exam is normal. Corneal scraping is performed and sent for gram stain and culture. The gram stain reveals gram-positive cocci.

After initiating a topical antibiotic for 48 hours, the patient returns to your clinic with symptoms improving. He asks whether there anything else that can be added to his therapy to improve his vision. How should you counsel this patient?

A. There is nothing else that can be done.
B. We can add a topical corticosteroid to decrease the risk of corneal ring; however, it may increase the risk of corneal perforation.
   ~~ can add a topical corticosteroid to decrease the risk of cor~
       ~wever, it may increase the risk of a rise in IOP to betw~

D. We can add a topical corticosteroid, which may decrease the risk of corneal scarring; however, a study known as SCUT showed there was no improvement in visual acuity at 3 months.

Suggested Answer

This bacterial corneal ulcer can be categorized as small, shallow, and noncentral. According to the results of SCUT, adding topical corticosteroids in this
patient will not produce any benefit in visual acuity at 3 months (option D).

References

1. Srinivasan M, Mascarenhas J, Rajaraman R, et al.; Steroids for Corneal Ulcers Trial
Group. Corticosteroids for bacterial keratitis: the Steroids for Corneal Ulcers Trial
(SCUT). *Arch Ophthalmol.* 2012;130(2):143–50.
2. Srinivasan M, Mascarenhas J, Rajaraman R, et al.; Steroids for Corneal Ulcers Trial
Group. The Steroids for Corneal Ulcers Trial: study design and baseline characteristics. *Arch Ophthalmol.* 2012;130(2):151–7.
3. Srinivasan M, Mascarenhas J, Rajaraman R, et al.; Steroids for Corneal Ulcers Trial
Group. The steroids for corneal ulcers trial (SCUT): secondary 12-month clinical
outcomes of a randomized controlled trial. *Am J Ophthalmol.* 2014;157(2):327–33.

4

Topical Natamycin Versus Voriconazole for Fungal Corneal Ulcer[*]

Mycotic Ulcer Treatment Trial (MUTT)

Natamycin treatment was associated with significantly better clinical and microbiological outcomes than voriconazole treatment for smear-positive filamentous fungal keratitis, with much of the difference attributed to improved results in *Fusarium* cases.

—The Mutt Group[1]

Research Question: Does topical treatment with natamycin give better clinical and microbiological outcomes than voriconazole for smear-positive filamentous fungal keratitis?[1]

Funding: National Eye Institute, National Institutes of Health; That Man May See; Harper/Inglis Trust; South Asia Research Foundation; Research to Prevent Blindness.

Year Study Began: 2010.

Year Study Published: 2013.

Study Location: 3 centers in South India.

---

[*] Basic and Clinical Science Course, Section 8. *External Disease and Cornea.* San Francisco: American Academy of Ophthalmology; 2018–2019: 276.

Who Was Studied: Patients, 16 years of age and older, with smear-positive filamentary fungal corneal ulcer and baseline visual acuity of 20/40 to 20/400.

Who Was Excluded: Patients were excluded if they had evidence of ocular coinfection, active bilateral ulcers, visual acuity less than 20/200 in the fellow eye, or impending perforation.

How Many Patients: 323.

Study Overview: The Mycotic Ulcer Treatment Trial (MUTT) was a randomized, active comparator–controlled, double-masked, clinical trial (Figure 4.1).[1]

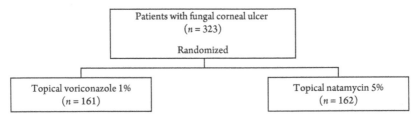

Figure 4.1. Summary of MUTT.

Study Intervention: Study participants were randomized to receive topical voriconazole 1% or topical natamycin 5%, applied to the affected eye every hour while awake for 1 week/until reepithelialization, then every 2 hours while awake until 3 weeks from enrollment.

Follow-Up: 3 months.

Endpoints: The primary outcome was best spectacle-corrected visual acuity (BSCVA) at 3 months. Secondary outcomes included BSCVA at 3 weeks, infiltrate or scar size at 3 weeks and 3 months, time to reepithelialization, microbiological cure at 6 days (±1 day), and corneal perforation and/or therapeutic penetrating keratoplasty (TPK).

RESULTS

- More than half of the enrolled patients had *Fusarium* (40%) or *Aspergillus* (17%).
- Natamycin-treated cases had significantly better 3-month BSCVA than voriconazole-treated cases ($P = .006$).

- At 3 weeks the BCVA was 1.1 lines poorer in the voriconazole group.
- At 3 months the BCVA was 1.8 lines poorer in the voriconazole group.
- Natamycin-treated cases were less likely to have perforation or require TPK (odds ratio [OR] = 0.42; P = .009).
  - 34 perforations occurred in the voriconazole arm and 18 in the natamycin arm.
- *Fusarium* cases fared better with natamycin than with voriconazole.
  - The *Fusarium* patients in the natamycin arm read 4.1 lines better than the voriconazole arm (P < .001 for difference in BSCVA). BCVA was noted to be similar between the two arms in non-*Fusarium* infected patients.
  - In the *Fusarium* patients the OR for perforation on natamycin, compared to voriconazole, was 0.06 (P < .001). In non-*Fusarium* patients the OR was 1.08.
- A higher percentage of patient randomized to the natamycin arm were culture negative at 6 days. Again, this finding was most pronounced in the *Fusarium* subgroup.
- Reepithelization time and 3-month infiltrate or scar size did not significantly differ between the two treatments. However, in subgroup analysis, *Fusarium* cases healed more rapidly with natamycin and had significantly smaller scars at 3 months.

Criticisms and Limitations: All patients in this study were enrolled in South India, and most infections were the result of agricultural exposure/trauma and not contact lens wear. Patients in other regions may have different risk factors, so the results of this study may not be generalizable.

This study compared only topical monotherapies and did not assess whether topical voriconazole could add benefit when used in conjunction with natamycin. Also, the cost of medications was not factored into this study (topical voriconazole may be more expensive than topical natamycin, which is an important factor in low-income countries).

Voriconazole showed good efficacy in in vitro studies; the lack of superior efficacy in this study may be attributable to intermittent drug dosing of topical voriconazole, resulting in intervals of subtherapeutic drug levels.

Other Relevant Studies and Information:

- A randomized clinical trial comparing the efficacy of topical voriconazole and topical natamycin with that of intrastromal voriconazole and topical

natamycin in patients with recalcitrant fungal keratitis showed no
beneficial effect of intrastromal injections over topical therapy.[2]

- The Mycotic Ulcer Treatment Trial II (MUTT II), a double-masked,
  placebo-controlled, randomized clinical trial conducted in India and
  Nepal, in which patients with smear-positive filamentous fungal ulcers
  and visual acuity of 20/400 or worse were randomized to receive oral
  voriconazole for 20 days versus oral placebo, in addition to topical
  antifungal eyedrops, showed no benefit to adding oral voriconazole to
  topical antifungal agents (despite the fact that oral voriconazole exhibits
  excellent ocular penetration).[3]
  - Overall, no difference in the rate of corneal perforation or the need
    for TPK was determined for oral voriconazole versus placebo (hazard
    ratio, 0.82; $P = .29$).
- A Cochrane review of 12 trials concluded that there was evidence that
  natamycin is more effective than voriconazole in the treatment of fungal
  ulcers, noting that the trials were of variable quality and were generally
  underpowered.[4]

Summary and Implications: Topical natamycin is superior to topical voriconazole in filamentous fungal keratitis. Monotherapy with topical voriconazole
cannot be recommended for filamentous fungal keratitis.

CLINICAL CASE: A YOUNG MAN WITH A FUNGAL CORNEAL ULCER

Case History
A 24-year-old white man who works as a gardener presents to your clinic with
a 3-day history of pain and blurring of vision in the right eye. His visual acuity
is 20/400 in the right eye, and slit lamp exam shows a white, fluffy-appearing
corneal infiltrate. A corneal scraping demonstrates a filamentous fungal or-
ganism. How would you proceed with treatment of this patient based on the
findings in MUTT?

A. Topical voriconazole 1 gtt hourly as a monotherapy.
B. Topical natamycin 1 gtt hourly as a monotherapy.
C. Topical natamycin and voriconazole 1 gtt hourly as topical therapy.
D. Topic amphotericin 1 gtt hourly as a monotherapy.

Suggested Answer
Option B.

References

1. Prajna NV, Krishnan T, Mascarenhas J, et al.; Mycotic Ulcer Treatment Trial Group. The mycotic ulcer treatment trial: a randomized trial comparing natamycin vs voriconazole. *JAMA Ophthalmol.* 2013;131(4):422–9.
2. Sharma N, Chacko J, Velpandian T, et al.. Comparative evaluation of topical versus intrastromal voriconazole as an adjunct to natamycin in recalcitrant fungal keratitis. *Ophthalmology.* 2013;120(4):677–81.
3. Prajna NV, Krishnan T, Rajaraman R, et al.; Mycotic Ulcer Treatment Trial II Group. Effect of oral voriconazole on fungal keratitis in the Mycotic Ulcer Treatment Trial II: a randomized clinical trial. *JAMA Ophthalmol.* 2016;134(12):1365–72.
4. FlorCruz NV, Evans JR. Medical interventions for fungal keratitis. *Database Syst Rev.* 2015;(4):CD004241.

5

Prevalence of Age-Related Lens Opacities in a Population*

The Beaver Dam Eye Study

Age-related lens opacities are common [in adults in the United States] and are a frequent cause of loss of vision. Overall, 17.3% had nuclear sclerosis more severe than level 3 in a 5-step scale of severity. Cortical opacities . . . were found in 16.3% of the population. Posterior subcapsular opacities occur in 6.0% of the population.

—Klein et al[1]

Research Question: What is the prevalence and severity of lens opacities in a rural community in the United States?[1]

Funding: National Eye Institute, National Institutes of Health.

Year Study Began: 1988.

Year Study Published: 1992.

Study Location: Wisconsin, United States.

Who Was Studied: Residents of Beaver Dam.

* Basic and Clinical Science Course, Section 11. *Lens and Cataract.* San Francisco: American Academy of Ophthalmology; 2018–2019: 6–7.

Who Was Excluded: No-one was excluded; however, rates in 87 participants who were housebound or in nursing homes were not reported because only 13 had gradable lens photographs.

How Many Participants: 4,926.

Study Overview: The Beaver Dam Eye Study was a population-based cohort study designed to collect information on the prevalence and incidence of age-related cataract, macular degeneration, and diabetic retinopathy. A total of 5,925 adults between the ages of 43 and 84 years were identified by a private phone census; 4,926 agreed to participate and be examined (56% women; 64% in the 75+ age group). The results of the baseline examination for cataract are reported in this paper.[1]

Study Intervention: None—this was a cross-sectional study. Direct slit-lamp and retroillumination photographs of the lens of each eye were taken through dilated pupils and graded using standardized methods.[2] Slit-lamp photographs were graded for severity of nuclear sclerosis (NS) on a 5-point scale; lens color was graded separately. Retroilluminated photographs were used to estimate the area involved by cortical and posterior subcapsular (PSC) opacities using a circular measuring grid with 9 segments. Less than 2% of eyes had no gradable photographs.

Follow-Up: None—this was a cross-sectional study.

Endpoints: Frequency (%) of lens opacities by type, age group, and sex.

RESULTS

- NS more severe than level 3 in a 5-step scale of severity was found in 17.3% of right eyes.
  - There was no significant difference in severity between right and left eyes.
  - Men had a lower prevalence of more severe NS at all ages.
- Rates of yellowing of the lens (right eye) in women ranged from 1.5% for those between 43 and 54 years of age, to 74.1% for those 75 years of age or older.
  - Rates of yellowing were lower for men.
- Cortical opacities involving at least 5% of the lens were found in 16.3% of the population.

- • Cortical opacities were more common in women ($P < .002$).
  - • The inferior nasal sectors of the lens were more involved than the others.
- • White anterior cortical opacities were found in 9.7% of right eyes.
- • PSC opacities occurred in 6.0% of the population, most commonly in the central circle.
- • Overall, approximately 15% of people between 43 and 54 years of age had early cataract (defined as NS level 3 and/or cortical opacity involving 5%–24% of the lens and/or PSC opacity involving 5%–24% of the lens).
- • In the 75+age group, visually significant cataract (defined as any cataract, early or late, in the presence of best corrected visual acuity (BCVA) of 20/32 or worse in the affected eye) was found in 45.9% (worse eye) in women and 38.8% (worse eye) in men.
  - • In the 43–54 year age group, visually significant cataract was found in 2.6% (worse eye) in women and 0.4% (worse eye) in men. (See Table 5.1.)

Table 5.1. FREQUENCY (%) OF LENS OPACITIES BY TYPE AND AGE GROUP

Age (years)	NS >level 3/5 (right eye)	Cortical	White anterior cortical (right eye)	PSC	Any (right eye) Early[†]	Late[‡]
43–54	<0.5*	1.5	1.8	1.6	11.1	0.5
55–64	4*	n/a	4.1	n/a	32.7	5.5
65–74	19*	n/a	13.8	n/a	50.3	24.0
75+	45*	42.4	31.8	14.3	36.6	52.2
Total	17.3	16.3	9.7	6.0	30.8	15.3

NS, nuclear sclerosis; PSC, posterior subcapsular; n/a, not available
[†] NS level 3 and/or cortical 5%–24% and/or PSC 5%–24%
[‡] NS level 4–5 and/or cortical ≥25% and/or PSC ≥25%
* estimated from Figure 2 in paper

Criticisms and Limitations: Whether these prevalence estimates can be generalized to the entire US adult population depends on whether the adult population of Beaver Dam, Wisconsin (and in particular the sample examined in this study), is representative of the general US adult population. This cannot be determined, as no sociodemographic or health information is given.

Other Relevant Studies and Information:

- The Salisbury Eye Evaluation Project examined a representative sample of 2,520 community-dwelling persons aged 65–84 years in Salisbury, Maryland, 26.4% of whom were African American. Overall, 55% of Caucasians and 68% of American Americans had any lens opacity.[3]
  - The odds of having cortical opacities were 4.0 times greater among African Americans than among Caucasians.
  - Caucasians were significantly more likely to have nuclear opacities (odds ratio = 2.1) and PSC opacities (odds ratio = 2.5).
- Using pooled cataract prevalence data from 7 population-based studies among populations relevant to the United States which used a standardized system of cataract grading, Congdon et al estimated that 17.2% of Americans older than 40 years had cataract in either eye.[4]
  - Women have a significantly higher age-adjusted prevalence of cataract than men in the United States (odds ratio = 1.37).
- In a follow-up study of the Beaver Dam Eye Study cohort, over a 15-year interval the cumulative incidence of nuclear cataract was 29.7%; of cortical cataract, 22.9%; and of PSC, 8.4%.[5]

Summary and Implications: Lens opacities are common in adults in the United States, and the numbers are increasing as the population ages. Prevalence data are important for providing for social and healthcare needs and planning for future services.

CLINICAL CASE: EARLY LENS OPACITY IN A YOUNG MAN

Case History

A 45-year-old man presents with a 6-month history of hazy vision in his left eye, worse in bright light. He is concerned about losing his eyesight. He has no history of eye disease or trauma, no significant past medical history, has never smoked, and takes no regular medications. He has worked outdoors since the age of 15 in various occupations such as landscaping, roofing, and construction. His mother developed a retinal detachment at age 53, which was treated surgically; however, the visual result was poor as she had waited several months after onset before going to an ophthalmologist. The patient is worried that he has developed something similar. On examination his visual acuity is 20/25 in the right eye and 20/40 in the left eye. Slit-lamp examination shows early PSC cataract in both eyes, more so in the left eye. No other abnormalities are found. He asks how common cataracts are. How would you respond?

A. Cataracts are most common in the middle life age range (43–54 years of age).
B. PSC cataracts tend to be the most common type of cataract.
C. Right eyes tends to develop a cataract more rapidly than left eyes.
D. In the Beaver Dam Eye Study, approximately 15% of adults between 43 and 54 years of age had early cataract.

Suggested Answer

You reassure him that there is no sign of retinal detachment in either eye, and explain that his symptoms are caused by early cataract formation. When he expresses surprise at this—he was under the impression that cataract only developed in the elderly—you tell him that, while this is generally true, in one survey (the Beaver Dam Eye Study) approximately 15% of those between 43 and 54 years of age had early cataract (option D). He feels better and promises to return in 1 year for a follow-up exam. In the meantime, you advise him to wear a wide-brimmed hat and sunglasses with UV protection when outside for extended periods.

References

1. Klein BE, Klein R, Linton KL. Prevalence of age-related lens opacities in a population: the Beaver Dam Eye Study. *Ophthalmology*. 1992;99(4):546–52.
2. Klein BEK, Klein R, Linton KLP, et al. Assessment of cataracts from photographs in the Beaver Dam Eye Study. *Ophthalmology*. 1990;97:1428–33.
3. West SK, Muñoz B, Schein OD, Duncan DD, Rubin GS. Racial differences in lens opacities: the Salisbury Eye Evaluation (SEE) project. *Am J Epidemiol*. 1998;148(11):1033–9.
4. Congdon N, Vingerling JR, Klein BE, et al.; Eye Diseases Prevalence Research Group. Prevalence of cataract and pseudophakia/aphakia among adults in the United States. *Arch Ophthalmol*. 2004;122(4):487–94.
5. Klein BE, Klein R, Lee KE, Gangnon RE. Incidence of age-related cataract over a 15-year interval the Beaver Dam Eye Study. *Ophthalmology*. 2008;115(3):477–82.

6

Risk Factors for Cataract*

The Lens Opacities Case-Control Study

Cataract is associated with low education, a nonprofessional occupation, intake of vitamins and iron, and body mass. Diabetes is a risk factor for all cataract types, except nuclear; use of oral steroids is associated with posterior subcapsular cataract and use of gout medications with mixed cataract.

—LESKE ET AL[1]

Research Question: What are the main risk factors associated with nuclear, cortical, and posterior subcapsular (PSC) lens opacities?[1]

Funding: National Eye Institute, National Institutes of Health.

Year Study Began: 1985.

Year Study Published: 1991.

Study Location: Boston, Massachusetts, Unites States.

* Basic and Clinical Science Course, Section 11. *Lens and Cataract.* San Francisco: American Academy of Ophthalmology; 2018–2019.

Who Was Studied: Cases and controls were general ophthalmology outpatients, aged 40–79 years, at the Massachusetts Eye and Ear Infirmary and the Brigham and Women's Hospital, Boston, Massachusetts (and resident in Massachusetts).

Who Was Excluded: Persons with diagnoses that precluded full pupillary dilatation (to at least 6 mm), lens evaluation at the slit lamp, or lens photography were ineligible, as were patients with other types of cataract or eye pathology causing a loss of visual acuity.

How Many Participants: 1,380.

Study Overview: The Lens Opacities Case-Control Study was designed to have four case groups (nuclear, cortical, PSC, or mixed cataract) and one control group (no cataract) (Figure 6.1).[1]

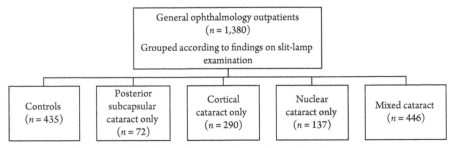

Figure 6.1. Summary of the Lens Opacities Case-Control study.

Study Intervention: None—this was a case-control study. The type and degree of lens opacification were graded at the slit lamp and from lens photographs following the protocol of the Lens Opacities Classification System I (LOCS I) that was developed for use in this study.[2,3] This system, which is based on standard photographs, provides ordinal scores of the degree of opacification separately for the nuclear (N_0, N_1, or N_2), cortical (C_0, C_{1a}, C_{1b}, or C_2), and PSC (P_0, P_1, or P_2) regions of the lens. Information was collected on the following groups of hypothesized risk factors: (1) nutritional factors (including intake of proteins, vitamins, and calcium; body mass index); (2) medical and medication history (including diabetes and cardiovascular diseases; use of oral steroids, antihyperuricemics, aspirin, smoking, and alcohol); (3) personal characteristics (including education and occupation, race, and iris color); and (4) environmental and other factors (including sunlight exposure, myopia and use of eyeglasses, and family history). Each of the risk factors evaluated in the study was identified a priori.

Follow-Up: None—this was a case-control study.

Endpoints: Odds ratios (ORs) for different cataract types by hypothesized risk factors.

RESULTS

- Modifiable factors associated with a lower risk of cataract:
  - Regular use of multivitamin supplements decreased risk for all cataract types (OR = 0.63).
  - Dietary intake of riboflavin, vitamin C, vitamin E, and carotene was protective for cortical, nuclear, and mixed cataract; intake of niacin, thiamine, and iron also decreased risk.
  - Body mass index was associated with lower risk of nuclear cataract (OR = 0.76).
  - Occupational exposure to sunlight was associated with lower risk of nuclear cataract (OR = 0.61).
- Modifiable factors associated with an increased risk of cataract:
  - Diabetes increased the risk of PSC, cortical, and mixed cataracts (OR = 1.56).
  - Current smoking increased the risk of nuclear cataract (OR = 1.68).
  - Oral steroid therapy increased PSC cataract risk (OR = 5.83).
  - Gout medications increased risk of mixed cataract (OR = 2.48).
  - Use of eyeglasses by age 20 years (an indicator of myopia) increased risk of mixed cataract (OR = 1.44).
- Other associations:
  - Females (OR = 1.51) and nonwhites (OR = 2.03) were at increased risk only for cortical cataract.
  - A nonprofessional occupation was associated with increased risk for nuclear cataract (OR = 1.96).
  - Low education increased risk for all cataract types (OR = 1.46).

Criticisms and Limitations: In any case-control study, possible selection and information (misclassification) biases must always be carefully considered during both the design and conduct of the study. In this study selection bias was minimized by selecting cases and controls from outpatients visiting the same general eye services, an approach that increased their comparability on socioeconomic, demographic, healthcare utilization, and other factors. Ascertainment bias could exist for diabetes because diabetics consult ophthalmologists more frequently than nondiabetics; such bias appears unlikely, since diabetes frequency was not increased in all the case groups. Knowledge of risk factor status is also unlikely to have affected patient selection for the study, because (1) a detailed protocol for case and control selection was followed, (2) the recruiting staff was unaware of the specific factors under study, and (3) most risk factors were determined after participation. Misclassification of persons into the case and control groups was minimized by using a simple and reproducible system of lens classification; in addition, more than half of the classifications were performed by one examiner. Interviewer bias was minimized by following a standardized protocol and format; the interviewer was also unaware of the case or control status of the participant and of the specific study hypotheses. Recall bias seems unlikely, since the case-control differences were seen only for those self-reported factors and were specific (except for multivitamin use) for some cataract types only. Furthermore, the results of the physician verification of medical information (such as medication use and diabetes) showed no difference in the results for cases and controls.

Other Relevant Studies and Information:

- The LOCS I, developed for use in this study, was later thought to span too large a range of cataractous change in too few steps to serve investigators interested in measuring the rate of cataract growth.[2,3] The LOCS II allowed grading into more categories.[4] This has evolved into LOCS III, with narrowed scaling intervals, allowing small changes in cataract severity to be observed.[5]
- The many risk factors identified to date can be grouped into individual factors, lifestyle factors, diet, systemic medical problems, ocular disorders, trauma (blunt and penetrating), and radiation (ionizing, infrared, and microwave).[6-9]
- In India, case-control studies showed a strong association between risk of cataract and remembered episodes of dehydrational crises from severe cholera-like diarrheal disease.[10,11]
  - People exposed to one or more remembered episodes of severe dehydrational crisis from severe diarrhea have, on average, a 3–4 times higher risk of cataract.
- Use of certain drugs can increase the risk of cataract formation: systemic, topical or inhaled corticosteroids, phenothiazines, miotics, amiodarone, and statins.
  - A meta-analysis of 7 studies of antidepressants use and risk of cataract found that the combined ORs of cataract for selective serotonin reuptake inhibitors (SSRIs), serotonin noradrenalin reuptake

inhibitors (SNRIs), and tricyclic antidepressants (TCAs) were 1.12, 1.13, and 1.19, respectively.[12]

Summary and Implications: Results from the Lens Opacities Case-Control Study and other studies suggest a multifactorial etiology in cataractogenesis, where personal, nutritional, medical, and other exposures accelerate lens opacification, perhaps through the common pathway of oxidative damage. A potential for modifying cataract risk is suggested by the associations with nutritional intake and use of multivitamin supplements. The study also suggests a role for other potentially modifiable factors, such as use of some medications and smoking.

QUESTION: RISK FACTORS FOR CATARACT

Which one of the following is the most important risk factor associated with cataract?

A. Diabetes.
B. Corticosteroid use.
C. Age.
D. Microwave radiation.
E. Genetic factors.

Answer:

The correct answer is C. The most important risk factor associated with cataract is age; almost everyone living long enough will develop cataract.

References

1. Leske MC, Chylack LT Jr, Wu SY. The lens opacities case-control study: risk factors for cataract. *Arch Ophthalmol.* 1991;109(2):244–51.
2. Chylack LT Jr, Leske MC, Sperduto R, Khu P, McCarthy D. Lens opacities classification system. *Arch Ophthalmol.* 1988;106(3):330–4.
3. Leske MC, Chylack LT Jr, Sperduto R, Khu P, Wu SY, McCarthy D. Evaluation of a lens opacities classification system. *Arch Ophthalmol.* 1988;106(3):327–9.
4. Chylack LT Jr, Leske MC, McCarthy D, Khu P, Kashiwagi T, Sperduto R. Lens opacities classification system II (LOCS II). *Arch Ophthalmol.* 1989;107(7):991–7.
5. Chylack LT Jr, Wolfe JK, Singer DM, et al. The Lens Opacities Classification Systems (III): the Longitudinal Study of Cataract Study Group. *Arch Ophthalmol.* 1993;111(6):831–6.

6. Chang JR, Koo E, Agrón E, et al; Age-Related Eye Disease Study Group. Risk factors associated with incident cataracts and cataract surgery in the Age-Related Eye Disease Study (AREDS): AREDS report number 32. *Ophthalmology*. 2011;118(11):2113–9.

7. Gupta VB, Rajagopala M, Ravishankar B. Etiopathogenesis of cataract: an appraisal. *Indian J Ophthalmol*. 2014;62(2):103–10.

8. Lam D, Rao SK, Ratra V, et al. *Cataract. Nat Rev Dis Primers*. 2015;1:15014.

9. Liu YC, Wilkins M, Kim T, Malyugin B, Mehta JS. Cataracts. Lancet. 2017;390(10094):600–12.

10. Minassian DC, Mehra V, Jones BR. Dehydrational crises from severe diarrhoea or heatstroke and risk of cataract. *Lancet*. 1984;1(8380):751–3.

11. Minassian DC, Mehra V, Verrey JD. Dehydrational crises: a major risk factor in blinding cataract. *Br J Ophthalmol*. 1989;73(2):100–5.

12. Fu Y, Dai Q, Zhu L, Wu S. Antidepressants use and risk of cataract development: a systematic review and meta-analysis. *BMC Ophthalmol*. 2018;18(1):31.

7

High-Dose Supplementation with Vitamins C and E and Beta Carotene for Age-Related Cataract and Vision Loss[*]

The Age-Related Eye Disease Study (AREDS)

Use of a high-dose formulation of vitamin C, vitamin E, and beta carotene in a relatively well-nourished older adult cohort had no apparent effect on the 7-year risk of development or progression of age-related lens opacities or visual acuity loss.

—AREDS RESEARCH GROUP[1]

Research Question: Does high-dose antioxidant formulation affect the development and progression of age-related lens opacities and visual acuity loss?[1]

Funding: National Eye Institute, National Institutes of Health, and Bausch & Lomb Inc, Rochester, NY.

Year Study Began: 1992.

Year Study Published: 2001.

Study Location: 11 centers in the United States.

---

[*] Basic and Clinical Science Course, Section 11. *Lens and Cataract*. San Francisco: American Academy of Ophthalmology; 2018–2019: 7–8, 63–64.

Who Was Studied: The Age-Related Eye Disease Study (AREDS) was a multi-center study of the natural history of age-related cataract and macular degeneration (AMD), including a clinical trial component consisting of 2 trials generally sharing 1 pool of participants (Figure 7.1).[2] The ocular eligibility criteria were largely determined by requirements for the study of AMD. Except for the requirement that the media be sufficiently clear in a study eye to obtain quality stereoscopic fundus photographs of the macula, lens opacity status itself was not considered in selecting participants. All participants had a best-corrected visual acuity of 20/32 or better (visual acuity score of ≥74 letters on the Early Treatment Diabetic Retinopathy Study (ETDRS) logMAR chart) in at least 1 eye. Participants were aged 55 to 80 years; persons aged 55 to 59 years were enrolled only if eligible for AMD Categories 3 and 4.

Who Was Excluded: Potential participants were excluded for illness or disorders (such as a history of cancer with a poor 7-year prognosis, major cardiovascular or cerebrovascular event within the last year, or hemachromatosis) that would make long-term follow-up or compliance with the study protocol unlikely or difficult.

How Many Participants: 4,629 in the cataract trial.

Study Overview: The aim of the randomized clinical trial was to evaluate the effect of the antioxidants vitamin C, vitamin E, and beta carotene in combination on the development or progression of age-related lens opacities, and the effect of both the antioxidants and high doses of zinc on the progression to advanced AMD.

Study Intervention: The 4 treatment interventions were double masked and given as an oral total daily supplementation of antioxidants (500 mg of vitamin C, 400 IU of vitamin E, and 15 mg of beta carotene) or zinc (80 mg of zinc as zinc oxide, 2 mg of copper as cupric oxide to prevent potential anemia), or the combination of antioxidants and zinc, or placebo. Participants supplementing with any of the study medication ingredients prior to randomization agreed to permanently stop using those supplements during the run-in period and take Centrum (Whitehall-Robins Healthcare, Madison, NJ), a multivitamin and mineral supplement with recommended daily allowance (RDA)–level dosages, provided by the study.

Follow-Up: Participants were followed for an average of 6.3 years.

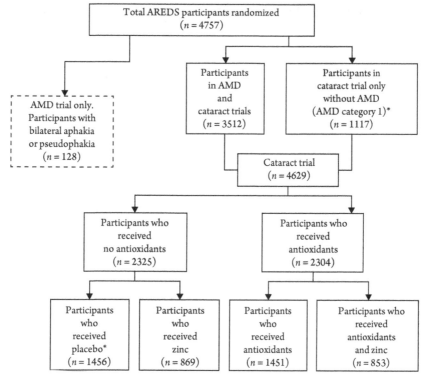

Figure 7.1. Summary of the AREDS.

Endpoints: Primary outcomes were (1) an increase from baseline in nuclear, cortical, or posterior subcapsular (PSC) opacity grades or cataract surgery, and (2) at least moderate visual acuity loss from baseline ($\geq$15 letters).

RESULTS

- No statistically significant effect of the antioxidant formulation was seen on the development or progression of age-related lens opacities (odds ratio = 0.97, P = .55).
- There was no statistically significant effect of treatment in reducing the risk of progression for any of the 3 lens opacity types or for cataract surgery.
- For the 1,117 participants with no AMD at baseline, no statistically significant difference was noted between treatment groups for at least moderate visual acuity loss.

Criticisms and Limitations: All AREDS participants were 55 years or older at enrollment in the study, and the median age was 68 years. At baseline 15% of the participants already had a nuclear grade of at least 4.0 U (on a scale of 0.9–6.1), 52% had some cortical opacities, and 10% had some PSC opacities. It is possible, even likely, that cataracts had probably already started to develop in many participants, even for those with no clinically apparent lens opacities. It may be that, for many, the AREDS intervention was started too late in the process for it to be effective.

The ability to reliably detect change using serial photographs taken at yearly intervals could have been affected by factors such as changes in the characteristics of the film available for purchase, the film development processes, and aging of the photographic equipment.

Fifty-five percent of the AREDS participants were taking dietary supplements of a multivitamin or at least 1 of the ingredients in the AREDS formulation prior to joining the study. The statistical power of the study to test its primary hypothesis about high doses of the study ingredients might have been reduced to the extent that prior use or the continued use of recommended daily allowance–type doses of these nutrients or other nutrients in the Study Intervention affected the risk of cataract development.

Other Relevant Studies and Information:

- A randomized, double-masked, placebo-controlled clinical trial involving 1,193 subjects aged 55 to 80 years with early or no cataract (the Vitamin E, Cataract and Age-Related Maculopathy Trial) found that natural vitamin E given for 4 years at a dose of 500 IU daily did not reduce the incidence of or progression of nuclear, cortical, or posterior subcapsular cataracts.[3]
- A randomized, double-masked, placebo-controlled clinical trial involving 1,020 participants 55 to 75 years old with early or no cataract (the Clinical Trial of Nutritional Supplements and Age-Related Cataract) found that, over an average follow-up period of 9 years (+/- 2.4 years), a daily tablet of a multivitamin/mineral formulation reduced the risk of a prespecified increase from baseline in nuclear cataract. but had no effect on cortical opacities, moderate visual acuity loss, or cataract surgery.[4]
  - The daily multivitamin/mineral formulation doubled the risk of a prespecified increase from baseline in posterior subcapsular cataract (PSC).
- A 2012 Cochrane Database systematic review and meta-analysis of 9 randomized controlled trials (RCTs) involving 117,272 individuals

concluded: "There is no evidence from RCTs that supplementation with antioxidant vitamins (beta-carotene, vitamin C or vitamin E) prevents or slows the progression of age-related cataract. We do not recommend any further studies to examine the role of antioxidant vitamins beta-carotene, vitamin C and vitamin E in preventing or slowing the progression of age-related cataract."[5]

Summary and Implications: High-dose supplementation with vitamins having antioxidant characteristics (vitamin C, vitamin E, and beta carotene) does not affect the development or progression of age-related lens opacities. However, a possible role for other micronutrients with or without antioxidant properties remain unanswered.

CLINICAL CASE: AN ELDERLY MAN WITH EARLY CATARACT IN BOTH EYES

Case History
A 69-year-old man complains of mild blurring of vision in both eyes, slightly worse in the left eye. He is a regular cigarette smoker (averaging 12 cigarettes per day), has no past medical history of note, and does not take any regular medications. Both parents had cataract surgery in their late-70s. On examination, visual acuities were 20/30 in the right eye and 20/60 in the left eye. Slit-lamp exam showed early PSC in both eyes. Nothing of note was found on fundoscopy. The patient has read on the Internet that daily multivitamins can slow the progression of cataracts and wants your advice. What should you tell him?

A. Vitamins containing antioxidants decrease the rate of cataract formation.
B. Vitamins containing antioxidants may actually increase the rate of cataract formation.
C. Vitamins containing antioxidants have not been proven to affect the rate of cataract formation.
D. Vitamins containing antioxidants have not been proven to affect the rate of cataract formation but zinc supplements have been proven to decrease cataract formation.

Suggested Answer

Based on the results of the AREDS study (AREDS report no. 9) and the most recent Cochrane database systematic review and meta-analysis, you inform him that there is currently no good evidence that antioxidant vitamins (such as vitamin C, vitamin E, and beta carotene) slow the progression of age-related lens opacities (option C). The most important action he can take is to stop smoking, and you refer him to the local tobacco cessation clinic. You also recommend that he wear a wide-brimmed hat and sunglasses with UV protection when outside for extended periods.

References

1. Age-Related Eye Disease Study Research Group. A randomized, placebo-controlled, clinical trial of high-dose supplementation with vitamins C and E and beta carotene for age-related cataract and vision loss: AREDS report no. 9. *Arch Ophthalmol.* 2001;119(10):1439–52.

2. The Age-Related Eye Disease Study Research Group. The Age-Related Eye Disease Study (AREDS): design implications: AREDS Report No. 1. *Control Clin Trials.* 1999;20:573–600.

3. McNeil JJ, Robman L, Tikellis G, Sinclair MI, McCarty CA, Taylor HR. Vitamin E supplementation and cataract: randomized controlled trial. *Ophthalmology.* 2004;111(1):75–84.

4. Clinical Trial of Nutritional Supplements and Age-Related Cataract Study Group, Maraini G, Williams SL, Sperduto RD, et al. A randomized, double-masked, placebo-controlled clinical trial of multivitamin supplementation for age-related lens opacities. Clinical trial of nutritional supplements and age-related cataract report no. 3. *Ophthalmology.* 2008;115(4):599–607.e1.

5. Mathew MC, Ervin AM, Tao J, Davis RM. Antioxidant vitamin supplementation for preventing and slowing the progression of age-related cataract. *Cochrane Database Syst Rev.* 2012;(6):CD004567.

8

Routine Preoperative Medical Testing Before Cataract Surgery*

Study of Medical Testing for Cataract Surgery

> Routine medical testing before cataract surgery does not measurably increase the safety of the surgery.
>
> —Schein et al[1]

Research Question: Does routine medical testing before cataract surgery reduce the rate of complications during the perioperative period?[1]

Funding: The Agency for Health Care Policy and Research.

Year Study Began: 1995.

Year Study Published: 2000.

Study Location: 9 clinical centers in the United States.

Who Was Studied: Patients scheduled to undergo elective cataract surgery.

Who Was Excluded: Patients were excluded from the study if they were less than 50 years old, were to receive general anesthesia, had a history of myocardial infarction within the preceding 3 months, or had undergone any preoperative medical testing during the 28 days before enrollment.

* Basic and Clinical Science Course, Section 1. *Update on General Medicine*. San Francisco: American Academy of Ophthalmology; 2018–2019: 284.

How Many Participants: 19,557 operations (18,189 patients).

Study Overview: See Figure 8.1.

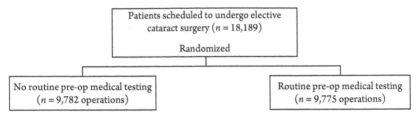

Figure 8.1. Summary of the Study of Medical Testing for Cataract Surgery.

Study Intervention: Patients whose operations were randomly assigned to the routine-testing group were given a letter and study brochure to take to the healthcare provider who was to perform the preoperative medical assessment, requesting that a 12-lead electrocardiogram, complete blood count, and measurements of serum electrolytes, urea nitrogen, creatinine, and glucose be obtained. If the patient's operation was randomly assigned to the no-testing group, the letter requested that no preoperative testing be performed, unless the patient presented with a new or worsening medical problem that would warrant medical evaluation with testing even if surgery were not planned.

Follow-Up: Adverse medical events and interventions on the day of surgery and during the seven days after surgery were recorded.

Endpoints: The rates of intraoperative and postoperative adverse events and the overall rate of complications (intraoperative and postoperative adverse events combined). The adverse events used in the study included myocardial infarction or ischemia, congestive heart failure, cardiac arrhythmia, hypertension, hypotension, stroke or transient ischemic attack, respiratory failure, bronchospasm, oxygen desaturation, hypoglycemia, diabetic ketoacidosis, and nonketotic hyperosmolar syndrome.

RESULTS

- The overall rate of complications (intraoperative and postoperative adverse events combined) was the same in the two groups (31.3 events per 1,000 operations).

- There were no significant differences between the no-testing group and the testing group in the rates of intraoperative adverse events (19.2 and 19.7, respectively, per 1,000 operations)
- There were no significant differences between the no-testing group and the testing group in the rates of postoperative adverse events (12.6 and 12.1 per 1,000 operations).
- The types of medical events were similar in the groups, with the exception of bronchospasm, which occurred more frequently both intraoperatively and postoperatively in the no-testing group.
- Overall, treatment for hypertension and arrhythmia (principally bradycardia) accounted for 61% of the events in the no-testing group and 68% of the events in the routine-testing group.

Criticisms and Limitations: Almost 6% of patients crossed over from their allocated group. Crossover to preoperative testing occurred more frequently among sicker patients whose operations were randomly assigned to the no-testing group than among healthier patients. The differential health status of crossover patients could have biased the results by reducing the adverse event rate in the no testing group. With this in mind, the authors preformed an intention-to-treat analysis, rather than a per-protocol analysis, thus obtaining an unbiased comparison.

It is assumed that all participants in both groups had optimal assessment and care before surgery, but this is not stated.

Other Relevant Studies and Information:

- In a randomized clinical trial of 1,025 patients undergoing scheduled cataract surgery, routine medical testing before surgery did not reduce the rate of ocular surgical complications and did not influence visual acuity outcome.[2]
  - The cumulative rate of ocular surgical complications was 20.5% in the routine-testing group and 19.3% in the selective-testing group ($P = .624$).
  - The preoperative and the postoperative best corrected visual acuity were similar in both groups.
- A Cochrane review published in 2012 concluded that routine preoperative medical testing did not reduce the risk of intraoperative (OR = 1.02) or postoperative medical adverse events (OR = 0.96) when compared to selective or no testing.[3]

- In a retrospective cohort study of 968 consecutive patients undergoing cataract surgery there were no perioperative major cardiovascular events.[4] Hypertension occurred in 319 (33%) patients, accounting for 79.7% of all adverse events.
  - Preoperative evaluation resulted in a lower hypertension rate after adjustment for propensity score (OR = 0.6); no effects were observed on posterior capsule rupture and emergency visits/hospitalization within 7 days of surgery.
  - Eighty-nine patients (9.3%) had an initial systolic pressure ≥180 mm Hg, which was not associated with higher risk of posterior capsule rupture ($P = .158$) or postoperative adverse events ($P = .902$).

Summary and Implications: Routine preoperative medical testing before cataract surgery does not reduce the risk of intraoperative or postoperative medical adverse events when compared to selective or no testing, nor does it reduce the rate of ocular surgical complications (such as posterior capsule rupture) or influence visual acuity outcome. Preoperative clinical assessment by a physician at least 7 days before surgery is a more logical and efficient approach. Tests should be ordered only when indicated by the history or findings on physical examination.

CLINICAL CASE: PREOPERATIVE MEDICAL TESTING BEFORE CATARACT SURGERY

Case History

A 73-year-old man is referred for evaluation of a visually significant cataract. He has a past medical history of diabetes with a recent HgbA1c of 7.2%, has a history of myocardial infarction 4 years ago, and is currently on clopidogrel. In preparation for surgery under monitored anesthesia care (MAC), what is the best way to proceed with his preoperative assessment?

A. A complete history and physical exam along with complete blood count (CBC), chemistry, EKG, and chest X-ray.
B. A complete history and physical exam along with CBC and chemistry.
C. A complete history and physical exam along with an EKG.
D. A complete history and physical exam without further testing unless strong evidence suggests an acute or worsening medical condition.

Suggested Answer

Option D. Patients undergoing routine elective cataract surgery who are not undergoing anesthesia do not benefit from routine preoperative medical testing such as chemistry, CBC, EKG, or chest X-ray. They should have a thorough systemic evaluation to ensure they do not have any new or unstable medical condition, and testing should be ordered as needed based on the results of this evaluation.

References

1. Schein OD, Katz J, Bass EB, et al. The value of routine preoperative medical testing before cataract surgery. Study of Medical Testing for Cataract Surgery. *N Engl J Med*. 2000;342(3):168–75.
2. Nascimento MA, Lira RP, Soares PH, Spessatto N, Kara-José N, Arieta CE. Are routine preoperative medical tests needed with cataract surgery? Study of visual acuity outcome. *Curr Eye Res*. 2004;28(4):285–90.
3. Keay L, Lindsley K, Tielsch J, Katz J, Schein O. Routine preoperative medical testing for cataract surgery. *Cochrane Database Syst Rev*. 2012;(3):CD007293.
4. Alboim C, Kliemann RB, Soares LE, Ferreira MM, Polanczyk CA, Biolo A. The impact of preoperative evaluation on perioperative events in patients undergoing cataract surgery: a cohort study. *Eye (Lond)*. 2016;30(12):1614–622.

9

Prophylaxis of Postoperative Endophthalmitis Following Cataract Surgery*

ESCRS Endophthalmitis Study

> The results presented here [also] indicate that with the prophylactic use of intracameral cefuroxime, the incidence rate [of endophthalmitis] can be reduced to a level below 0.08%.
>
> —ESCRS ENDOPHTHALMITIS STUDY GROUP[1]

Research Question: Does antibiotic prophylaxis reduce the incidence of postoperative endophthalmitis after cataract surgery? What are the main risk factors associated with endophthalmitis after cataract surgery?[1]

Funding: European Society of Cataract & Refractive Surgeons (ESCRS), Dublin, Ireland; Santen GmbH, Germering, Germany.

Year Study Began: 2003.

Year Study Published: 2007.

Study Location: 24 hospitals in 9 European countries.

Who Was Studied: Patients undergoing phacoemulsification cataract surgery with placement of an intraocular lens (IOL) as a single procedure without additional surgery.

* Basic and Clinical Science Course, Section 11. *Lens and Cataract*. San Francisco: American Academy of Ophthalmology; 2018–2019: 162–163.

Who Was Excluded: Patients who were allergic to penicillins and cephalosporins, in long-term nursing homes, younger than 18 years, and all groups severely "at risk" for infection, such as those with severe atopic keratoconjunctivitis or active blepharitis, were excluded.

How Many Participants: 16,603 patients.

Study Overview: This was a prospective, randomized, partially masked, clinical trial using a 2 × 2 factorial design, with prophylactic intracameral cefuroxime and topical perioperative levofloxacin factors resulting in 4 treatment groups of approximately equal sizes (Figure 9.1).[1,2]

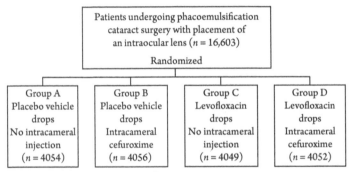

Figure 9.1. Summary of the ESCRS Endophthalmitis study.

Study Intervention: Group A received no perioperative antibiotic prophylaxis, Group B received the intracameral cefuroxime treatment (cefuroxime injected into the anterior chamber at the end of surgery as 1 mg in 0.1 mL normal saline) only, Group C received the topical levofloxacin treatment (levofloxacin 0.5% administered 1 drop 1 hour before surgery, 1 drop 30 minutes before surgery, and 3 drops at 5-minute intervals commencing immediately after surgery) only, and Group D received both intracameral cefuroxime and topical levofloxacin treatments. The levofloxacin treatment was masked; with patients receiving placebo or antibiotic drops from bottles supplied as part of the study. The use of cefuroxime was not masked; surgeons were requested to give patients who had been randomly allocated to Groups B and D the intracameral injection at the end of surgery.

All patients received povidone–iodine 5% drops (Betadine) into the conjunctival sac and onto the cornea for a minimum of 3 minutes before surgery, and all patients were requested to use levofloxacin 0.5% eyedrops (Oftaquix) 4 times daily for 6 days starting the day after surgery.

Follow-Up: 27 months (study terminated early when the Data Monitoring Committee was informed that there were significant findings on the prophylactic use for 1 of the 2 antibiotics).

Endpoints: A diagnosis of presumed endophthalmitis was made for any patient presenting with pain or loss of vision thought to be due to infection. Samples of aqueous and vitreous were collected from these patients and investigated using Gram staining, culture, and polymerase chain reaction testing using nonspecific microbial primers. Any case in which at least 1 of these tests yielded a positive result was classified as proven infective endophthalmitis. The total endophthalmitis cases constituted these proven cases together with those identified by the clinicians but for which no positive proof of infection was found. Each unproven case was reviewed for evidence of toxic anterior segment syndrome (TASS) or noninfective uveitis.

RESULTS

- Twenty-nine patients presented with endophthalmitis, of whom 20 were classified as having proven infective endophthalmitis.
- The absence of an intracameral cefuroxime prophylactic regimen was associated with a nearly 5-fold increase in the risk for total postoperative endophthalmitis.
- The total case numbers and incidence rates (by intention-to-treat analysis) in each group were as follows:
  - Group A: Placebo vehicle drops/no intracameral injection: 14 (0.345%).
  - Group B: Placebo vehicle drops/intracameral cefuroxime 1 mg: 3 (0. 074%).
  - Group C: Levofloxacin drops 0.5%/no intracameral injection: 10 (0.247%).
  - Group D: Levofloxacin drops 0.5%/intracameral cefuroxime 1 mg: 2 (0.049%).
- The use of clear corneal incisions compared to scleral tunnels was associated with a nearly 6-fold increase in risk of endophthalmitis.
- The use of silicone intraocular lens optic material compared to acrylic was associated with a 3-fold increase in risk of endophthalmitis.
- The presence of surgical complications increased the risk for total endophthalmitis nearly 5-fold.
  - "Experienced" surgeons were twice as likely to participate in an endophthalmitis case. (See Table 9.1.)

Table 9.1. ESTIMATED ORs AND THE ASSOCIATED 95% CIs FROM THE FINAL
LOGISTIC REGRESSION MODELS OF THE RISK FACTORS FOR TOTAL AND PROVEN
ENDOPHTHALMITIS CASES

Risk Factor		Total Endophthalmitis Cases		Proven Endophthalmitis Cases	
		OR (95% CI)	*p* Value	OR (95% CI)	*p* Value
No cefuroxime injection	vs. cefuroxime injection	4.92 (1.87–12.9)	.001	5.86 (1.72–20.0)	.005
Placebo eyedrops	vs. levofloxacin eyedrops	1.41 (0.67–2.95)	.368	1.51 (0.62–3.7)	.368
Clear corneal incision	vs. scleral tunnel	5.88 (1.34–25.9)	.019	7.43 (0.97–57.0)	.054
Silicone IOL	vs. acrylic IOL	3.13 (1.47–6.67)	.003	4.10 (1.66–10.1)	.002
Any surgical complication	vs. no surgical complication	4.95 (1.68–14.6)	.004	—	—

CI = confidence interval; IOL = intraocular lens; OR = odds ratio

Criticisms and Limitations: The study was not fully masked. Surgeons were requested to give the intracameral injection at the end of surgery only to patients who had been randomly allocated to Groups B and D. However, full masking would have been unethical. In any case, it is very unlikely that the lack of full masking resulted in any bias.

No data are given on the composition of the 4 groups, so it is impossible to say whether they are balanced with respect to sociodemographic and clinical covariates and comorbidities.

Other Relevant Studies and Information:

- In a retrospective review of 31,386 cataract surgeries, the intracameral injection of cefuroxime reduced the rate of postoperative infectious endophthalmitis in cataract surgery significantly.[3]
  - The incidence of endophthalmitis decreased from 1.38 per 1,000 patients in the period 2002–2009 (during which subconjunctival mezlocillin and postoperative gentamicin eye drops were given) to 0.44 per 1,000 patients in the period 2009–2013 (during which intracameral cefuroxime moxifloxacin drops were given).
- In a retrospective review of 8,239 cataract surgeries, the incidence of postoperative endophthalmitis decreased approximately 8-fold (from

0.49% to 0.06%) following the introduction of intracameral cefuroxime following cataract surgery.[4]

- A Cochrane review published in 2017 concluded: "High-certainty evidence shows that injection with cefuroxime with or without topical levofloxacin lowers the chance of endophthalmitis after surgery, and there is moderate-certainty evidence to suggest that using antibiotic eye drops in addition to antibiotic injection probably lowers the chance of endophthalmitis compared with using injections or eye drops alone."[5]

Summary and Implications: Use of intracameral cefuroxime at the end of surgery reduces the occurrence of postoperative endophthalmitis. To reduce the risk further, consideration should be given to avoiding silicone IOLs and using a scleral tunnel incision rather than a clear corneal incision.

CLINICAL CASE: ANTIBIOTIC PROPHYLAXIS AFTER CATARACT SURGERY

Case History
A 75-year-old man is scheduled for phacoemulsification cataract surgery with placement of an intraocular lens (IOL) in the right eye. He is concerned about the possibility of postoperative infection in the eye and poor visual result. Ten years previously a similar operation on the left eye was complicated by postoperative endophthalmitis, which was treated by administration of broad-spectrum antibiotics and dexamethasone injection into the vitreous cavity. The final corrected visual acuity was 6/60. According to the ESCRS Endophthalmitis Study, which perioperative consideration is MOST likely to reduce his risk of endophthalmitis associated with cataract surgery on this second eye?

A. Use of a clear corneal incision.
B. Use of a silicone IOL.
C. Use of intracameral cefuroxime injection.
D. Use of preoperative levofloxacin drops.

Suggested Answer
Option C. After reviewing the surgical notes from 10 years ago, you determine that standard practice at that time was to give subconjunctival administration of mezlocillin and postoperative antibiotic eye drops (gentamicin) without intracameral injection at the end of cataract surgery. You explain to the patient

that, based on the results of the ESCRS endophthalmitis study, standard practice now is to give an intracameral injection of cefuroxime at the end of surgery,
along with topical antibiotic drops. Although the risk of postoperative infection is never completely eliminated, this practice has been shown to reduce the
rate of postoperative endophthalmitis to less than 0.08% (8 in 10,000), which
is extremely low. To risk the risk further, you will use a scleral tunnel incision
and an acrylic IOL. The patient is reassured.

References

1. Prophylaxis of postoperative endophthalmitis following cataract surgery: results of
   the ESCRS multicenter study and identification of risk factors. Endophthalmitis
   Study Group, European Society of Cataract & Refractive Surgeons. *J Cataract Refract
   Surg*. 2007;33(6):978–88.
2. Seal DV, Barry P, Gettinby G, et al. ESCRS study of prophylaxis of postoperative
   endophthalmitis after cataract surgery; case for a European multicenter study; the
   ESCRS Endophthalmitis Study Group. *J Cataract Refract Surg*. 2006;32:396–406.
3. Röck T, Bramkamp M, Bartz-Schmidt KU, et al. [Using intracameral cefuroxime
   reduces postoperative endophthalmitis rate: 5 years experience at the University Eye
   Hospital Tübingen]. *Klin Monbl Augenheilkd*. 2014;231(10):1023–8.
4. Rahman N, Murphy CC. Impact of intracameral cefuroxime on the incidence of
   postoperative endophthalmitis following cataract surgery in Ireland. *Ir J Med Sci*.
   2015;184(2):395–8.
5. Gower EW, Lindsley K, Tulenko SE, Nanji AA, Leyngold I, McDonnell PJ.
   Perioperative antibiotics for prevention of acute endophthalmitis after cataract surgery. *Cochrane Database Syst Rev*. 2017;2:CD006364.

10

The Relationship Between Optic Disc Area and Open-Angle Glaucoma*

The Baltimore Eye Survey

> Disc area is a weak risk factor for open angle glaucoma.
> —QUIGLEY ET AL[1]

Research Question: Do eyes with larger optic disc areas have a higher risk for developing open-angle glaucoma (OAG)?[1]

Funding: United States Public Health Service.

Year Study Began: 1984.

Year Study Published: 1999.

Study Location: Baltimore, Maryland, United States.

Who Was Studied: Noninstitutionalized adults older than 40 years of age residing in East Baltimore, Maryland.

Who Was Excluded: Patients were excluded if they were medically unhealthy and could not participate.

---

* Basic and Clinical Science Course, Section 10. *Glaucoma*. San Francisco: American Academy of Ophthalmology, 2018–2019: 81–83.

How Many Participants: 5,308.

Study Overview: The Baltimore Eye Survey was a population-based survey of the prevalence of ocular disorders in East Baltimore, Maryland.[1,2] A total of 5,308 individuals underwent a detailed screening eye examination, including automated perimetry (using a Humphrey Field Analyzer), optic disc photography, and intraocular pressure (IOP) measurement (measured by applanation tonometry). Participants with best corrected visual acuity less than 20/30 in either eye, IOP greater than 21 mm Hg in either eye, visual field loss, abnormal optic disc characteristics on photographic review, or a history of glaucoma underwent a second examination by another ophthalmologist and visual field testing using Goldmann perimetry.

Study Intervention: None; this was a population-based survey. In the first analysis, one eye (the eye with the largest disc area) from each patient with glaucoma was compared with those of subjects without glaucoma. The study defined OAG as a reproducible visual field loss (on two Goldmann perimetry tests) and a compatible optic disc appearance (judged by a masked glaucoma specialist). No IOP criteria were used in the definition of glaucoma. In the second analysis among patients with OAG, disc area was correlated with IOP.

Follow-Up: None; this was a cross-sectional study.

Endpoints: Standardized optic disc measurements were corrected for spherical equivalent refraction error. The IOP level was the median of 3 measurements.

RESULTS

- Of the 5,308 individuals who underwent initial screening/testing, 161 (3.03%) were identified as having OAG.
  - Usable optic disc images were obtained for 3,593 persons, including 75 with OAG and 3,518 without glaucoma.
- Optic disc area was slightly larger, on average, among those with OAG.
  - Disc area was 2.87 +/- 0.59 mm² among those without glaucoma and 3.11 +/- 0.61 mm² among those with OAG.
  - After adjusting for age, race, and gender, the difference in disc area was not statistically significant ($P = 0.06$).
- Among the 75 patients with OAG, disc area was not significantly related to IOP level after adjusting for age, race, and gender ($P = .77$).

- There was no statistically significant difference in disc area between black and white patients with OAG ($P = .55$).

Criticisms and Limitations: This was a population-based study conducted in a single area within Baltimore, Maryland. Although the racial breakdown of the participants was roughly balanced, it could be difficult to extrapolate these findings data to a different community.

The patients with usable disc photos were on average younger than those with unusable photos. Furthermore, in patients with severe visual field loss only 4% had usable imaging. This likely missed more advanced cases of glaucoma that could have potentially had a different distribution of disc areas.

Other Relevant Studies and Information:

- The Baltimore Eye Survey published several papers looking at risk factors for OAG.[2,3] These studies identified race, intraocular pressure, systemic hypertension, and family history as important risk factors for developing glaucoma.
- Established and important risk factors for primary OAG now include low ocular perfusion pressure, type 2 diabetes, myopia, and thin central cornea in addition to age, race/ethnicity, IOP, and family history of glaucoma.[4]

Summary and Implications: There was no statistically significant difference in overall disc area between patients with OAG and control subjects, although there was a trend toward having larger discs in patients with OAG.

CLINICAL CASE: RISK FACTORS FOR OPEN-ANGLE GLAUCOMA

Case History

You suspect that a patient has open-angle glaucoma based on visual field findings and the appearance of the optic discs. You are wondering whether there are any other risk factors that the patient may have that help stratify this patient's risk of having/developing OAG. Based on the Baltimore Eye Survey and subsequent studies, which statement is true?

A. Larger optic disc area was a statistically significant risk for OAG in the Baltimore Eye Survey.
B. Family history is an important risk factor for developing glaucoma..
C. Caucasian race was a statistically significant risk factor for OAG in the Baltimore Eye Survey.
D. The correlation between larger disc area and higher IOP was statistically significant in the Baltimore Eye Survey.

Suggested Answer
Option B.

References

1. Quigley HA, Varma R, Tielsch JM, Katz J, Sommer A, Gilbert D. The relationship between optic disc area and open-angle glaucoma: the Baltimore Eye Survey. *J Glaucoma*. 1999;8:347–52.
2. Tielsch JM, Sommer A, Witt K, Katz J, Royall RM. Blindness and visual impairment in an American urban population: the Baltimore Eye Survey. *Arch Ophthalmol*. 1990;108:286–90.
3. Tielsch JM, Sommer A, Katz J, Royall RM, Quigley HA, Javitt J. Racial variations in the prevalence of primary open-angle glaucoma: the Baltimore Eye Survey. *JAMA*. 1991;266:369–74.
4. Prum BE Jr, Rosenberg LF, Gedde SJ, Mansberger SL, Stein JD, Moroi SE, Herndon LW Jr, Lim MC, Williams RD. Primary Open-Angle Glaucoma Preferred Practice Pattern(®) Guidelines. *Ophthalmology*. 2016;123(1):P41–P111.

11

Is Argon Laser Trabeculoplasty Equivalent to Topical Medication as an Initial Treatment for Primary Open-Angle Glaucoma?*

The Glaucoma Laser Trial (GLT)

> It appears that ALT is at least as good as, if not better than, starting with medications, because, in the short term, ALT provides good pressure control and has the advantage of postponing and/or reducing the inconvenience, nuisance, and side effects associated with taking medications.
>
> —GLT RESEARCH GROUP[1]

Research Question: Is the efficacy and safety of argon laser trabeculoplasty (ALT) equivalent to treatment with topical medication for controlling intraocular pressure (IOP) in patients with newly diagnosed, previously untreated primary open-angle glaucoma (POAG)?[1]

Funding: National Eye Institute, National Institutes of Health.

Year of Data Collection: 1984.

Year of Publication: 1990.

* Basic and Clinical Science Course, Section 10. *Glaucoma*. San Francisco: American Academy of Ophthalmology; 2018–2019: 188.

Study Location: 8 clinics in the United States.

Who Was Studied: Patients, 35 years of age and older, newly diagnosed with POAG with IOP in both eyes ≥22 mm Hg on 2 consecutive visits no more than 2 months apart and a glaucomatous visual field defect in at least one eye (or disc abnormalities in the presence of extremely elevated lOP), plus best corrected visual acuity (BCVA)better than 20/70 in both eyes.

Who Was Excluded: Patients with a history of non-POAG glaucoma; history of IOP-lowering medication (topical or systemic) within the prior 6 months; severe paracentral or global visual field defect; previous ocular surgery (including laser and corneal surgery); a severely scarred angle sufficient to preclude ALT; or evidence of diabetic retinopathy, neovascularization, or rubeosis iridis.

How Many Patients: 271 (542 eyes).

Study Overview: This was a randomized, single-blind, controlled clinical trial (Figure 11.1).[1]

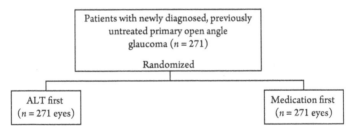

Figure 11.1. Summary of the GLT.

Study Intervention: To avoid having all eyes with higher lOP assigned to the same treatment group, patients were assigned to one of two strata: the stratum with right eye high IOP (and left eye low IOP) or the stratum with left eye high IOP (and right eye low IOP). Patients with equal lOP in both eyes were assigned to one of these strata at random. The ALT-first eyes received two sessions of ALT 4 weeks apart. The medication-first eyes were started on a stepped medication regimen, starting with topical timolol maleate 0.5% twice daily. In both arms, if the target IOP was not reached or there was deterioration of the visual fields or worsening of the optic disc appearance, and/or if the patient suffered adverse effects of the treatment regimen, then treatment was escalated through a stepped regimen: dipivefrin (step 2), low-dose pilocarpine (step 3), high-dose pilocarpine (step 4), timolol with high-dose pilocarpine (step 5), and dipivefrin with high-dose pilocarpine (step 6). If treatment eyes did not reach target IOP following the stepped regimen, the eyes were released from the study protocol and could be treated according to the specialist's discretion (although carbonic anhydrase inhibitors were discouraged). Eyes receiving intraocular surgery were also released from the study protocol.

Follow-Up: 2 years.

Endpoints: The primary endpoint was the time to prescription of two or more medications simultaneously. Secondary endpoints included change in visual field, change in optic disc appearance, change in IOP, and change in visual acuity.

RESULTS

- In the first 3 months, ALT-first eyes had an initial IOP lowering of 9 mm Hg compared to 7 mm Hg in the medication-first eyes.
  - Thereafter, the mean IOP for ALT-first eyes was approximately 2 mm Hg below that for the medication-first eyes.
- At 2 years, 44% of ALT-first eyes were deemed adequately controlled with ALT alone, compared to 30% of medication-first eyes.
  - Seventy percent of ALT-first eyes were controlled by ALT, or ALT and timolol.
  - Eighty-nine percent of ALT-first eyes and 66% of medication-first eyes were controlled with the stepped medication regimen ($P < .001$).
- At all times, more medication-first eyes than ALT-first eyes required the addition of another glaucoma medication for IOP control.
- Visual acuity remained stable in both groups at all follow-up times.
- Visual field changes were similar in the two groups.
- Peripheral anterior synechiae (PAS) developed more frequently in ALT-first eyes (34%) compared to medication-first eyes (3%).
  - Eyes with PAS required less medication for control of IOP compared to those without PAS, but this was not statistically significant. These eyes continued to have similar, or better, IOP reductions and stable visual fields when compared to eyes without PAS.
- Systemic and ocular side effects were similar in the two treatment arms.

Criticisms and Limitations: This was one of the first clinical trials to assess ALT versus medication as initial treatment for POAG. The crossover effect of timolol (i.e., timolol use in the medication-first eye could have an effect in the ALT-first eye) was judged to be small (estimated to be 0.5 mm Hg). Given the nature of glaucoma medication compliance, the authors could not be sure that medications were self-administered to the correct eye at the correct intervals; however, when questioned, the patients indicated that few mix-ups occurred.

The 2-year follow-up period was not really long enough to evaluate glaucomatous progression (changes in the visual field) between the two treatment arms. Also, the frequency of inconvenience and nuisance (of medication therapy) in the two groups—one of the main proposed advantages of using ALT first—was not reported.[2]

Patients in the GLT had to meet specific IOP requirements, be newly diagnosed, and have minimal visual field defect. The generalizability of the findings of this trial to a more general population of POAG patients (e.g., including previously treated patients) and more general methods of treatment, may be limited.

Other Relevant Studies and Information:

- Follow-up of 203 of the 271 patients who enrolled in the GLT (median duration of follow-up since diagnosis of POAG 7 years; maximum, 9 years) showed that the eyes treated initially with ALT had lower IOP and better visual field and optic disc status than their fellow eyes treated initially with topical medication.[3]
  - As compared to eyes initially treated with medication, eyes initially treated with ALT had 1.2 mm Hg greater reduction in IOP ($P < .001$) and 0.6 dB greater improvement in the visual field ($P < .001$).
  - The overall difference between eyes with regard to change in ratio of optic cup area to optic disc area was -0.01 ($P = .005$), which indicated slightly more deterioration for eyes initially treated with medication.
- Selective laser trabeculoplasty (SLT), which uses a Q-switched, frequency-doubled Nd:YAG laser, has increasingly been used to lower IOP in POAG and ocular hypertensive patients.[4,5] SLT requires much less energy and appears to have the same efficacy as ALT.
- In recent years, newer laser trabeculoplasty technologies have been introduced that appear to have similar efficacy when compared with the SLT or ALT. In addition, they potentially offer a more favorable safety profile with fewer complications, such as postlaser inflammation and IOP spikes. Further large-scale studies are necessary to evaluate the long-term benefits of these newer forms of laser trabeculoplasty.[5,6]

Summary and Implications: Initial treatment of POAG with ALT is an efficacious and safe alternative to medication therapy, particularly in patients where medical therapy is contraindicated or poor compliance is suspected. The initial use of ALT in the short term has the benefit of reducing nuisance, inconvenience, and systemic side effects of the topical glaucoma medication alternatives. At the conclusion of the extended follow-up study, those initially treated with laser trabeculoplasty had a clinical status similar to, or better than, the eyes treated initially with medication.

CLINICAL CASE: AN ELDERLY WOMAN WITH NEWLY DIAGNOSED OPEN-ANGLE GLAUCOMA

Case History

A 70-year-old African American woman presents to your clinic complaining of slowly decreasing vision and difficulty driving over the past 4 years. She describes difficulty seeing oncoming traffic on the left and right when stopped and difficulty changing lanes on the highway. She has long-standing memory deficits due to her progressive Alzheimer's disease, and has difficulty remembering to take her medications. On examination, her BCVA is 20/30 in both eyes, IOP is 26 mm Hg in both eyes, pupils are equal without relative afferent pupillary defect, and there is early cataract in both eyes. The cup-to-disc ratio is 0.65 bilaterally, and static field perimetry reveals a nasal step defect in both eyes. Her anterior and posterior segment exams are otherwise unremarkable. Gonioscopy reveals open angles in both eyes without visible scars. On follow-up examination 2 weeks later, IOP is 26 mm Hg in both eyes. Which regimen would you recommend as initial treatment of this patient's POAG?

A. Observation only with repeat IOP check in 3 months.
B. Topical timolol maleate 1 drop twice daily in both eyes.
C. Argon laser trabeculoplasty in both eyes.
D. Immediate trabeculectomy.

Suggested Answer

Given her progressive Alzheimer's disease, compliance with medical therapy is likely to be poor. The GLT found that initial treatment with ALT is at least as safe and efficacious as initial topical therapy with timolol and offers, in addition, the benefit of "decreased nuisance and inconvenience," compared to topical medications. Therefore, initial treatment with ALT (option C) would be recommended given her Alzheimer's disease.

References

1. The Glaucoma Laser Trial (GLT). 2. Results of argon laser trabeculoplasty versus topical medicines. The Glaucoma Laser Trial Research Group. *Ophthalmology.* 1990;97(11):1403–13.
2. Lichter PR. Practice implications of the Glaucoma Laser Trial. *Ophthalmol.* 1990;97(11):1401–2.
3. The Glaucoma Laser Trial (GLT) and glaucoma laser trial follow-up study: 7. Results. Glaucoma Laser Trial Research Group. *Am J Ophthalmol.* 1995;120(6):718–31.
4. Schlote T. [Status of selective laser trabeculoplasty (SLT)]. [Article in German; Abstract available in German from the publisher] *Klin Monbl Augenheilkd.* 2017;234(11):1362–71.
5. Garg A, Gazzard G. Selective laser trabeculoplasty: past, present, and future. *Eye (Lond).* 2018;32(5):863–76.
6. Tsang S, Cheng J, Lee JW. Developments in laser trabeculoplasty. *Br J Ophthalmol.* 2016;100(1):94–7.

12

Intraocular Pressure Reduction in the Treatment of Normal-Tension Glaucoma*

Collaborative Normal-Tension Glaucoma Study (CNTGS)

> The favorable effect of intraocular pressure reduction on progression of visual change in normal-tension glaucoma was only found when the impact of cataracts on visual field progression, produced largely by surgery, was removed.
>
> —CNTGS Group[1]

Research Question: What is the effectiveness of a 30% reduction in intraocular pressure (IOP) on visual field (VF) progression in eyes with normal-tension glaucoma?[1]

Funding: The Glaucoma Research Foundation (San Francisco, CA); Oxnard Foundation (Newport Beach, CA); Edward J. Daly Foundation (San Francisco, CA).

Year Study Began: 1984.

Year Study Published: 1998.

Study Location: 24 centers in the United States.

* Basic and Clinical Science Course, Section 10. *Glaucoma.* San Francisco: American Academy of Ophthalmology; 2018–2019: 87–88.

Who Was Studied: Patients, 21–89 years of age, with normal-tension glaucoma, with characteristic optic disc abnormalities and VF defects (based on 3 reliable baseline automated fields). After a 4-week washout of any existing glaucoma medication, patients had 10 baseline IOP readings, the median of which was required to be 20 mm Hg or less, and no single pressure reading could be greater than 24 mm Hg.

Who Was Excluded: Patients were excluded if they were taking systemic beta-blockers or clonidine, if they were unable to take a reliable VF, if they had a nonglaucomatous condition that might later affect VF, if they had previous laser treatment/ocular surgery (except strabismus)/cyclodestructive procedures, if they had field defects that could be attributable to nonglaucomatous conditions, if they had narrow/occludable angles, if they had corneal abnormalities, if best corrected visual acuity was less than 20/30, or if they had VFs too damaged to detect further progression reliably.

How Many Patients: 230 (145 eyes)

Study Overview: The Normal-Tension Glaucoma Trial was a randomized clinical trial (Figure 12.1).[1,2]

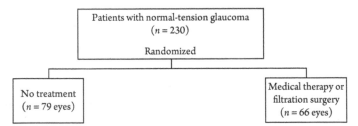

Figure 12.1. Summary of the CNTGS.

Study Intervention: One eye of each patient was randomized to the untreated control arm or the 30% IOP-reduced arm. The 30% IOP reduction group received either medical therapy or filtrating surgery to achieve the target IOP. Treatment was augmented as required to maintain the 30% reduction in IOP. In patients undergoing filtration surgery, a 20% IOP reduction was accepted without requiring the patient to undergo a second procedure, and no more than three surgical procedures were called for by the protocol in an effort to achieve the IOP goal. The goal was to achieve the 30% pressure lowering within 6 months (but the authors state that it often took longer). Neither eye could be treated with beta-blockers or adrenergic agonists because of possible cardiovascular and crossover effects that could confound the results.

Follow-Up: Not stated; approximately 7–8 years, judging from the figures.

Endpoints: The primary measures of outcome were VF progression (using 4-of-5 criteria) or change in the degree of glaucomatous optic disc damage.

RESULTS

- A smaller proportion (33.3%) in the IOP-reduced group developed VF progression compared to the untreated control group (39.2%), but this was not statistically significant.
  - The mean survival time before reaching a VF progression endpoint was 1,525 days for the control group and 1,796 days for the treated group ($P = .21$).
- Cataracts occurred in 11 (14%) of 79 control eyes and in 23 (35%) of 66 eyes in the treated group ($P = .0011$). Of these, 16 (48%) were among 33 surgically treated eyes and seven (25%) were among 28 eyes treated only with medication and laser trabeculoplasty ($P = .059$). The rate of development of cataracts in the untreated control subjects was significantly lower than in the surgically treated subgroup ($P = .0001$) but not statistically different from the rate in the medically treated subgroup ($P = .18$).
- After adjusting for the effect of cataract on visual acuity, a significantly smaller proportion (12.1%) in the IOP-reduced group developed VF progression compared to the untreated control group (26.6%) ($P = .0018$).
  - At 5 years, the survival analysis showed that 80% of patients in the treatment group had not met a VF progression endpoint, compared to 40% in the control group.
  - The mean survival time before reaching a VF progression endpoint was 1,476 days for the control subjects and 2,101 days for the treated group ($P = .0018$).

Criticisms and Limitations: Subgroup analysis by race and gender was not possible as the study numbers were too small. It is now recognized that female gender is a risk factor for progression in normal tension glaucoma, and that Asians tend to have slower glaucoma progression while African Americans tend to have faster progression.[2]

This study was carried out before the introduction of topical carbonic anhydrase inhibitors and prostaglandins which would have most likely reduced the number of surgical interventions that were particularly cataractogenic.

Foveal thresholds were used to determine whether the patient's VF was adversely affected by cataract rather than glaucoma. The assumption underlying this was that glaucoma should not affect central foveal thresholds, so if the decibel reading on a foveal threshold was lower between the baseline and the follow-up field, it was due to cataract. It is possible that some of these patients had glaucoma sufficiently advanced to have caused reduced foveal thresholds.

Other Relevant Studies and Information:

- In a companion paper, the CNTGS reported the results of an analysis in which the course of treated eyes was followed up from a new baseline established as soon as a 30% IOP reduction was stable, an average of 219 days after randomization. The results showed that reducing IOP by 30% decreased risk for glaucoma progression. It is important to note that a large percentage (65%) of those patients in the control group who did not get treatment never progressed. By setting a 30% pressure reduction goal in all patients with normal-tension glaucoma, a large number of people would be exposed to potential adverse effects from treatment for glaucoma that would have never progressed anyway.[3]
- Other risk factors for the progression of normal-tension glaucoma include female gender, migraine headache, and disc hemorrhages.[2] These risk factors help determine which patients are at highest risk of progression, perhaps needing more aggressive reduction of IOP.

Summary and Implications: Reducing the IOP of patients with normal tension glaucoma by 30% is beneficial to prevent progression of glaucomatous damage if the visual effects of cataracts are excluded from consideration. Because not all untreated patients progressed, the natural history of normal-tension glaucoma must be considered before embarking on IOP reduction with therapy apt to exacerbate cataract formation, unless normal tension glaucoma threatens serious visual loss.

CLINICAL CASE: AN ELDERLY WOMAN WITH NORMAL-TENSION GLAUCOMA

Case History

You have been following a 78-year-old white woman with normal-tension glaucoma. She is on two topical medications that have reduced her IOP about

10%–15% from its baseline. She appears to have worsening optic disc changes and visual field changes consistent with glaucoma. She would like to discuss treatment options and the necessity of treatment. How would you counsel her based on the CNTGS findings?

A. Reducing IOP by 30% is beneficial to prevent progression of normal-tension glaucoma if the visual effects from cataracts are excluded.
B. Reducing the IOP by 30% has no effect on the progression of normal-tension glaucoma in phakic patients.
C. Reducing the IOP by 30% does not outweigh the risks created by exacerbating cataract development in a patient with threats of serious vision loss from normal-tension glaucoma.
D. Reducing the IOP by 30% should only be considered in patients < 50 years of age who are unlikely to develop cataracts.

Suggested Answer
Option A. The CNTGS group concluded that reducing the IOP of patients with normal-tension glaucoma by 30% is beneficial to prevent the progression of glaucomatous damage if the visual effects of cataracts are excluded from consideration.

References

1. The effectiveness of intraocular pressure reduction in the treatment of normal-tension glaucoma. Collaborative Normal-Tension Glaucoma Study Group. *Am J Ophthalmol.* 1998;126(4):498–505.
2. Drance S, Anderson DR, Schulzer M; Collaborative Normal-Tension Glaucoma Study Group. Risk factors for progression of visual field abnormalities in normal-tension glaucoma. *Am J Ophthalmol.* 2001;131(6):699–708.
3. The Collaborative Normal Tension Glaucoma Study Group. Comparison of glaucomatous progression between untreated patients with normal-tension glaucoma and patients with therapeutically reduced intraocular pressures. *Am J Ophthalmol.* 1998;126(4):487–97.

13

The Relationship Between Control of Intraocular Pressure After Surgical Intervention for Glaucoma and Visual Field Deterioration*

The Advanced Glaucoma Intervention Study (AGIS)

Low intraocular pressure is associated with reduced progression of visual field defect, supporting evidence from earlier studies of a protective role for low intraocular pressure in visual field deterioration.

—THE AGIS INVESTIGATORS[1]

Research Question: Is the achievement of low levels of intraocular pressure (IOP) after surgical intervention associated with a slowing of visual field (VF) deterioration?[1]

Funding: National Eye Institute and the Office of Research on Minority Health, National Institutes of Health.

Year Study Began: 1988.

Year Study Published: 2000.

* Basic and Clinical Science Course, Section 10. *Glaucoma*. San Francisco: American Academy of Ophthalmology, 2018–2019: 114–115.

Study Location: 11 centers in the United States.

Who Was Studied: Patients, between the ages of 35 and 80 years, with open-angle glaucoma (OAG) that could no longer be adequately controlled by medications alone, despite maximum accepted and tolerated medical therapy. Eligible eyes had to meet specified criteria for combinations of consistently elevated IOP, glaucomatous VF defect, and/or optic disc rim deterioration;[2] for example, the minimum VF defect score was 1 and the maximum 16, on a scale of 0 (no defect) to 20 (end-stage).[3]

Who Was Excluded: Patients with a history of cataract removal.

How Many patients: 591 patients (789 eyes).

Study Overview: This paper (AGIS 7) reports the results of a pooled analysis of patients (eyes) enrolled in the Advanced Glaucoma Intervention Study (AGIS), disregarding their original randomized allocation.

The AGIS was a randomized clinical trial comparing two sequences of surgical treatments.[1,2] One sequence (ATT) began with argon laser trabeculoplasty (ALT), followed by trabeculectomy, should ALT fail to control the disease, and by a second trabeculectomy should the first trabeculectomy fail. The other sequence (TAT) began with trabeculectomy, followed by ALT should the trabeculectomy fail, and by a second trabeculectomy should ALT fail. Surgical interventions were supplemented by medical treatment with the goal of reducing IOP to less than 18 mm Hg. Both eyes of a patient were enrolled only if they were eligible simultaneously: one eye was randomly assigned to one of the sequences, and the fellow eye to the opposite sequence.

Study Intervention: None for this report. The entire cohort, regardless of original randomized allocation, was divided into groups for two separate analyses (Table 13.1). In the predictive analysis ($n = 738$ eyes followed up for at least 2 years), designed to determine whether the IOP during early follow-up is predictive of subsequent change in the VF defect score, IOP was averaged over the first three 6-month visits and the eye assigned to one of 3 categories. Then, for each subsequent 6-month follow-up visit, the mean in VF defect score was calculated. In the associative analysis ($n = 586$ eyes followed for at least 6 years), each eye was assigned to one of four categories based on the percent of visits over the first 6 years of follow-up for which an eye presented with IOP less than 18 mm Hg. Then, for each visit starting with the 6-month visit, the mean change in VF defect score was calculated.

Table 13.1. DEFINITIONS OF INTRAOCULAR PRESSURE GROUPS IN AGIS

Predictive Analysis IOP averaged over the first three 6-month visits	IOP group	Associative Analysis Percent of visits with IOP less than 18 mm Hg
<14 mm Hg	A	100
14–17.5 mm Hg	B	75 to <100
>17.5 mm Hg	C	50 to <75
	D	0 to <50

Follow-Up: Minimum 6 years.

Endpoints: Change in VF defect score measured from the preintervention reference (baseline) value.

RESULTS

- Both the predictive and associative analyses showed that low postintervention IOP is associated with reduced progression of VF defect. This association became stronger as follow-up lengthened.
  - Eyes with early average IOP greater than 17.5 mm Hg had an estimated worsening during subsequent follow-up that was 1 unit of VF defect score greater than eyes with average IOP less than 14 mm Hg ($P = .002$).
    - This amount of worsening was greater at 7 years (1.89 units; $P < .001$) than at 2 years (0.64 units; $P = .071$).
  - Eyes with 100% of visits with IOP less than 18 mm Hg over 6 years had mean changes from baseline in VF defect score close to zero during follow-up, whereas eyes with less than 50% of visits with IOP less than 18 mm Hg had an estimated worsening over follow-up of 0.63 units of VF defect score ($P = .083$).
    - This amount of worsening was greater at 7 years (1.93 units; $P < .001$) than at 2 years (0.25 units; $P = .572$).
- Patients with high IOP (>17.5 mm Hg) during follow-up were on average younger and had a higher prevalence of diabetes mellitus (DM) than patients with lower IOP.
- Eyes in the lowest IOP group experienced, on average, little VF deterioration during follow-up. This was most striking for eyes that maintained IOP less than 18 mm Hg at all study visits over 6 years. Although the average change in VF is close to zero, a proportion of eyes in

this group experienced VF loss despite having IOP at what is believed to be a safe level. In this low IOP group a worsening of four or more units of VF defect score from baseline was experienced by 13.1% of eyes at 2 years, 13.9% at 5 years, and 14.4% at 7 years.

Criticisms and Limitations: The analyses assessed IOP during follow-up without taking into account the glaucoma management employed to achieve IOP control. In addition, the IOP categories created for the predictive and associative analyses were not based on random allocation, thus introducing the possibility of confounding bias. There may be factors related to the progression of glaucoma that have not been accounted for.

Other Relevant Studies and Information:

- Post hoc analyses of the AGIS data generated many subsequent reports. Some of the main findings were:
  - Initial intervention with trabeculectomy retarded the progression of glaucoma more effectively in white than in black patients, whereas initial surgical intervention with ALT retarded the progression of glaucoma more effectively in black than in white patients.[4]
  - ALT failure was associated with younger age and higher preintervention IOP. Trabeculectomy failure was associated with younger age, higher preintervention IOP, DM, and one or more postoperative complications, particularly elevated IOP and marked inflammation.[5]
  - Risk factors for sustained decrease in VF were better baseline visual field in both treatment sequences, male gender, and worse baseline visual acuity in the ATT sequence, and DM in the TAT sequence. Risk factors for sustained decrease in visual acuity in both treatment sequences were better baseline visual acuity, older age, and less formal education.[6]
- Further investigation of the risk factors associated with VF progression in the AGIS cohort showed that both increasing age and greater IOP fluctuation increase the odds of VF progression by 30% for each 5-year increment in age and 1-mm-Hg increase in IOP fluctuation. The higher risk conferred by IOP fluctuation was consistently observed in eyes with and without a history of cataract extraction.[7]
  - Long-term IOP fluctuation is associated with VF progression in patients with low mean IOP but not in patients with high mean IOP.[8]

Summary and Implications: Low IOP is associated with reduced progression of VF defect, supporting evidence from earlier studies of a protective role for low IOP in visual field deterioration. However, maintaining IOP less than 18 mm Hg does not ensure the preservation of the VF.

CLINICAL CASE: A MIDDLE-AGED MAN WITH POORLY CONTROLLED GLAUCOMA

Case History
A 58-year-old American Indian man with a past medical history of DM and hypertension has been treated for glaucoma for over 12 years. He has already had ALT and a trabeculectomy in both eyes; however, his IOP is increasing again and is now ranging from 19 to 20 mm Hg on applanation measurements done during his past 3 visits. He has also had two consecutive worsening VFs despite being on maximal medical treatment. You are discussing with the patient your recommendation that he be evaluated for additional surgical treatment and you refer to the AGIS study in this discussion. With the findings of the AGIS in mind, which of the following statements concerning this patient is correct?

A. His multiple IOP measurements >18 mm Hg and his history of DM put him at high risk for glaucoma progression.
B. His history of ALT treatment, now considered outdated, may have worsened his glaucoma and, therefore, put him at high risk for glaucoma progression.
C. His race and his history of hypertension, along with his multiple IOP measurements > 18 mm Hg, put him at high risk for glaucoma progression.
D. Because he has already had an ALT, a repeat trabeculectomy will increase his risk of glaucoma progression.

Suggested Answer
Option A.

References

1. The Advanced Glaucoma Intervention Study (AGIS): 7. The relationship between control of intraocular pressure and visual field deterioration. The AGIS Investigators. *Am J Ophthalmol.* 2000;130(4):429–40.

2. Ederer F, Gaasterland DE, Sullivan EK; AGIS Investigators. The Advanced Glaucoma Intervention Study (AGIS): 1. Study design and methods and baseline characteristics of study patients. *Control Clin Trials.* 1994;15(4):299–325.

3. Advanced Glaucoma Intervention Study. 2. Visual field test scoring and reliability. *Ophthalmology.* 1994;101(8):1445–55.

4. AGIS Investigators. The Advanced Glaucoma Intervention Study (AGIS): 9. Comparison of glaucoma outcomes in black and white patients within treatment groups. *Am J Ophthalmol.* 2001;132(3):311–20.

5. AGIS Investigators. The Advanced Glaucoma Intervention Study (AGIS): 11. Risk factors for failure of trabeculectomy and argon laser trabeculoplasty. *Am J Ophthalmol.* 2002;134(4):481–98.

6. AGIS Investigators. The Advanced Glaucoma Intervention Study (AGIS): 12. Baseline risk factors for sustained loss of visual field and visual acuity in patients with advanced glaucoma. *Am J Ophthalmol.* 2002;134(4):499–512.

7. Nouri-Mahdavi K, Hoffman D, Coleman AL, et al.; Advanced Glaucoma Intervention Study. Predictive factors for glaucomatous visual field progression in the Advanced Glaucoma Intervention Study. *Ophthalmology.* 2004;111(9):1627–35.

8. Caprioli J, Coleman AL. Intraocular pressure fluctuation a risk factor for visual field progression at low intraocular pressures in the advanced glaucoma intervention study. *Ophthalmology.* 2008;115(7):1123–1129.e3.

14

Reduction of Intraocular Pressure and Glaucoma Progression[*]

Early Manifest Glaucoma Trial (EMGT)

The Early Manifest Glaucoma Trial is the first adequately powered randomized trial providing a long-term comparison of progression between treated and untreated patients with primary open-angle glaucoma, normal-tension glaucoma, and exfoliation glaucoma that shows a definite positive effect of IOP reduction.

—Heijl et al[1]

Research Question: In patients with newly detected, previously untreated primary open-angle glaucoma (POAG), does immediate institution of intraocular pressure (IOP)–lowering therapy reduce the risk of progression compared to delayed treatment or observation?[1]

Funding: National Eye Institute, National Institutes of Health; Swedish Medical Research Council, Stockholm.

Year Study Began: 1992.

Year Study Published: 2002.

[*] Basic and Clinical Science Course, Section 10. *Glaucoma*. San Francisco: American Academy of Ophthalmology; 2018–2019: 88, 113.

Study Location: Two centers in Sweden.

Who Was Studied: Patients, 50–80 years of age, with early, previously untreated POAG, pseudoexfoliation glaucoma, or normal-tension glaucoma in at least one eye, defined as having a visual field with reproducible defects and a mean deviation (MD) better than -4 dB, and a median IOP of 20 mm Hg.

Who Was Excluded: Patients were excluded if they had advanced visual field loss (MD less than or equal to 16 dB) or IOP greater than a mean of 30 mm Hg or a single reading of 35 mm Hg. Patients were also excluded if they had a significant cataract, visual acuity worse than 20/40, or were unable to perform reliable visual fields.

How Many Patients: 255.

Study Overview: This was a randomized, placebo-controlled clinical trial (Figure 14.1).[1,2]

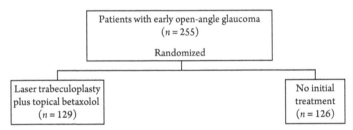

Figure 14.1. Summary of the EMGT.

Study Intervention: Patients were randomly allocated to either 360° argon laser trabeculoplasty (ALT) followed by topical betaxolol twice daily or no initial treatment. If patients in the observation group developed progression, they were offered immediate treatment (standard care). If pressure was not controlled on a single agent (> 25 mm Hg for two visits), nightly xalatan was added to the treatment regimen.

Follow-Up: Median follow-up was 6 years.

Endpoints: The primary measures of outcome were progression of either glaucomatous visual field defects or optic disc cupping. Definite visual field progression was defined as at least 3 test points showing significant progression, as compared with baseline, at the same locations on 3 consecutive glaucoma change probability maps. Optic disc progression was determined using flicker chronoscopy by masked evaluators.

RESULTS

- In the treatment group, the average reduction in IOP was 5.1 mm Hg (25%).
  - The reduction was larger (29%) in eyes with a baseline IOP of 21 mm Hg or greater than in eyes with a baseline IOP less than 21 mm Hg (18%).
  - In the control group, IOP values were unchanged (20.9 and 20.8 mm Hg at baseline and the 3-month visit, respectively), with small nonsignificant fluctuations thereafter (zero median change from 3 months to the end of the study).
- 53% of all patients showed progression of glaucoma.
  - Progression was less frequent in the treatment group (45%) than in controls (62%) ($P = .007$).
  - Progression occurred significantly later in treated patients (median 66 months) than in controls (median 48 months).
- The mean change in visual field loss from baseline to the end of follow-up, as expressed by the MD, was a worsening by 2.24 dB in the treatment group and 3.90 dB in the control group.
- Few systemic and ocular adverse effects (generally mild) were identified; however, both occurred more commonly in the treatment group.
  - There was a clear and significantly more rapid development of nuclear opacities (LOCS II gradings of 2 or higher) in the treatment group (approximately 16% vs. 4%, estimated from Figure 4 in the paper) ($P = .002$).
  - Cataract surgery was performed in 8 patients, 6 of whom were in the treatment group.
  - More patients died in the treatment group (15) than in the control group (7). This difference, although not statistically significant ($P = .08$), was observed within the first few years of follow-up.

Criticisms and Limitations: Almost all the patients were white, and from a single city; furthermore, most were healthy without significant ocular and medical comorbidities, which may limit the generalization of the findings to other populations.

The results apply only to persons with relatively early glaucoma and not to those with high IOP levels (>30 mm Hg) or advanced visual field loss. Also, the study did not include long-term follow-up of untreated patients beyond EMGT progression.

Other Relevant Studies and Information:

- In further analysis it was estimated that treatment halved the risk of progression (hazard ratio = 0.50).
  - Risk decreased about 10% with each millimeter mercury of IOP reduction from baseline; the higher (or lower) the IOP at follow-up, the higher (or lower) the risk.[3]
- IOP fluctuation was not found to be an independent factor for glaucoma progression, a finding that conflicts with some earlier reports—perhaps because analyses did not include postprogression IOP values, which would be biased toward larger fluctuations because of more intensive treatment.[4]
- Longer follow-up (median 8 years) showed that treatment and follow-up IOP continued to have a marked influence on progression, regardless of baseline IOP. Other significant factors were age, bilaterality, exfoliation, and disc hemorrhages, as previously determined. Lower systolic perfusion pressure, lower systolic blood pressure, and cardiovascular disease history emerged as new predictors, suggesting a vascular role in glaucoma progression. Another new factor was thinner central corneal thickness (CCT), with results possibly indicating a preferential CCT effect with higher IOP.[5]
- Evaluation of the relationship between IOP reduction attained with a fixed treatment protocol (360° laser trabeculoplasty and topical betaxolol eye drops twice daily, and no change in treatment as long as progression did not occur) found that the IOP reduction achieved depended very strongly on baseline untreated IOP levels. There seemed to be a lower threshold around 15 mm Hg, where therapy did not result in any reduction of IOP.[6]

Summary and Implications: IOP-lowering therapy offers a definitive benefit in patients with early glaucoma by delaying progression of glaucomatous optic neuropathy, especially in eyes with higher IOPs (>21 mm Hg) at baseline. Even modest reduction in IOP can help decrease the risk of progression. However, a large percentage of treated eyes still showed progression during follow-up. The progression of glaucomatous optic neuropathy is highly variable and difficult to predict for an individual patient.

CLINICAL CASE: A MIDDLE-AGED WOMAN WITH NEWLY DIAGNOSED OPEN-ANGLE GLAUCOMA

Case History

A 51-year-old woman with no significant past ocular history presents to you for routine examination. Her vision is 20/20 in both eyes without correction and she denies any ocular complaints. Her IOP is 25 mm Hg in the right eye and 24 mm Hg in the left eye by applanation; the remainder of her ocular examination is unremarkable with the exception of slight asymmetry of the cup-to-disc ratios, which were 0.6 in the right eye, with possible inferior thinning of the neuroretinal rim, and 0.5 in the left eye. Baseline measurement of the retinal nerve fiber layer optical coherence tomography shows borderline thinning inferiorly but is otherwise green in all quadrants. Automated perimetry shows a possible superior nasal step in the right eye. Repeat perimetry one month later confirms the nasal step with reliable indices. Based on the EMGT, what is the reduction in risk of glaucoma progression for this patient if her IOP is lowered to less than 21 mm Hg?

A. 40%.
B. 5%.
C. 10%.
D. 20%.

Suggested Answer

Option A. In the EMGT, risk decreased about 10% with each millimeter mercury of IOP reduction from baseline.

References

1. Heijl A, Leske MC, Bengtsson B, Hyman L, Bengtsson B, Hussein M; Early Manifest Glaucoma Trial Group. Reduction of intraocular pressure and glaucoma progression: results from the Early Manifest Glaucoma Trial. *Arch Ophthalmol.* 2002;120(10):1268–79.
2. Leske MC, Heijl A, Hyman L, Bengtsson B. Early Manifest Glaucoma Trial: design and baseline data. *Ophthalmology.* 1999;106(11):2144–53.
3. Leske MC, Heijl A, Hussein M, Bengtsson B, Hyman L, Komaroff E; Early Manifest Glaucoma Trial Group. Factors for glaucoma progression and the effect of treatment: the early manifest glaucoma trial. Arch Ophthalmol. 2003;121(1):48–56.

4. Bengtsson B, Leske MC, Hyman L, Heijl A; Early Manifest Glaucoma Trial Group. Fluctuation of intraocular pressure and glaucoma progression in the early manifest glaucoma trial. *Ophthalmology.* 2007;114(2):205–9.

5. Leske MC, Heijl A, Hyman L, Bengtsson B, Dong L, Yang Z; EMGT Group. Predictors of long-term progression in the early manifest glaucoma trial. *Ophthalmology.* 2007;114(11):1965–72.

6. Heijl A, Leske MC, Hyman L, Yang Z, Bengtsson B; EMGT Group. Intraocular pressure reduction with a fixed treatment protocol in the Early Manifest Glaucoma Trial. *Acta Ophthalmol.* 2011;89(8):749–54.

15

Topical Ocular Hypotensive Medication to Delay or Prevent the Onset of Primary Open-Angle Glaucoma[*]

The Ocular Hypertension Treatment Study (OHTS)

> Topical ocular hypotensive medication was effective in delaying or preventing POAG in eyes with ocular hypertension.
>
> —KASS ET AL[1]

Research Question: Does reducing intraocular pressure (IOP) in eyes with ocular hypertension (OHTN) reduce the risk of developing primary open-angle glaucoma (POAG)?[1]

Funding: National Eye Institute and the National Center on Minority Health and Health Disparities, National Institutes of Health; Merck Research Laboratories; Research to Prevent Blindness.

Year Study Began: 1994.

Year Study Published: 2002.

Study Location: 22 centers in the United States.

---

[*] Basic and Clinical Science Course, Section 10. *Glaucoma*. San Francisco: American Academy of Ophthalmology; 2018–2019: 80–83, 89–90, 112.

Who Was Studied: Patients 40–80 years of age with an IOP range of 24–32 mm Hg in one eye and 21–32 mm Hg in the other eye, open angles on gonioscopy, two normal visual fields, and normal optic discs. Recruitment was extended to ensure that 25% of participants were of African American origin.

Who Was Excluded: Patients were excluded if they had a visual acuity worse than 20/40 in either eye or previous intraocular surgery other than uncomplicated cataract extraction. Patients were also excluded if they had concurrent ocular diseases that could cause visual field loss or optic disc damage.

How Many Patients: 1,636.

Study Overview: The Ocular Hypertension Treatment Study (OHTS) was a randomized, open, placebo-controlled, clinical trial (Figure 15.1).[1,2]

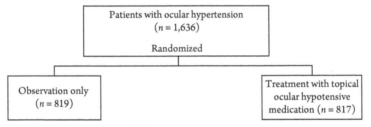

Figure 15.1. Summary of the OHTS.

Study Intervention: Patients were randomized to either observation or treatment with commercially available topical ocular hypotensive medication. The goal in the medication group was to reduce the IOP by 20% or more and to reach an IOP of 24 mm Hg or less.

Follow-Up: The median duration of follow-up was 72 months for African American participants and 78 months for other participants.

Endpoints: The primary outcome was development of POAG in one or both eyes as defined by reproducible visual field defects (3 consecutive fields) or optic disc deterioration on stereotactic optic disc photography attributable to POAG.

RESULTS

- The mean (± SD) baseline IOP of all participants in both groups was 24.9 (± 2.7) mm Hg.

- Patients in the intervention study arm had an average IOP reduction of 22.5% vs. an average IOP reduction of 4% in the observation arm.
  - The IOP reduction goal was met in both eyes in 87%, and in one eye in an additional 7%, of the scheduled follow-up visits completed by medication participants.
- In the medication group, 36 of the 817 participants developed POAG compared with 89 of 819 participants in the observation group.
  - At 60 months the cumulative probability of developing POAG was 4.4% in the treatment arm compared to 9.5% in the observation arm, resulting in a risk reduction of 60% over 5 years ($P < .0001$).
  - After adjusting for baseline age, visual field pattern standard deviation, vertical cup-disc ratio, IOP, and corneal thickness, the risk reduction was 66%.
- Treatment appeared to be less protective among self-identified African American participants.
  - POAG developed in 6.9% of African American participants in the medication group and 12.7% of African Americans in the observation group, a 46% risk reduction. This compared to a 66% risk reduction in other (mostly white) participants, although this difference was not statistically significant ($P = .26$).
- At 60 months, 2 or more topical medications were prescribed for 39.7% of the medication participants, and 3 or more medications were prescribed for 9.3% of participants.
- There was little evidence of increased systemic or ocular risk associated with ocular hypotensive medication.

Criticisms and Limitations: The OHTS used strict entry criteria and included generally healthy volunteers, which may limit the generalizability of the results.

The study treatment IOP reduction goal was set conservatively at 20% reduction, which may not have been low enough in patients with high-risk features or higher IOPs.[3] This may have overestimated the progression to glaucoma in treated eyes, as further IOP reduction could have potentially mitigated this risk. Furthermore, the medication regimen was not standardized and adherence to therapy was not monitored in the treatment group.

The parameters for detecting glaucomatous progression may have been too stringent, possibly resulting in a failure to detect more subtle presentations of early glaucomatous optic neuropathy. The true rate of conversion of patients to manifest glaucoma in both arms of the trial may have been underestimated.

Other Relevant Studies and Information:

- Further follow-up of the subgroup of African Americans in the OHTS, showed topical ocular hypotensive therapy was effective in delaying or preventing the onset of POAG in African American individuals who have OHTN.[4]
  - Among African American participants, 8.4% in the medication group developed POAG during the study compared with 16.1% in the observation group, a 50% risk reduction ($P =.02$).
- In a follow-up study to describe baseline demographic and clinical factors that predict which participants in the OHTS developed POAG, it was found that baseline age, vertical and horizontal cup-disc ratio, pattern standard deviation, and IOP were good predictors for the onset of POAG in the OHTS. Central corneal thickness was found to be a powerful predictor for the development of POAG.[5]
- To determine whether there is a penalty for delaying treatment, the OHTS participants in the original observation group (who received medication for a median of 5.5 years after a median of 7.5 years without treatment) were compared with the original medication group (who had a median time of treatment of 13.0 years).[6]
  - The cumulative proportion of participants in the original observation group who developed POAG at 13 years was 0.22, vs. 0.16 in the original medication group ($P = .009$).
  - Among participants at the highest third of baseline risk of developing POAG, the cumulative proportion that developed POAG was 0.40 in the original observation group and 0.28 in the original medication group.

Summary and Implications: Topical ocular hypotensive medication is effective in delaying or preventing the development of glaucomatous optic neuropathy in eyes with OHTN. However, not every patient with OHTN should be treated. Baseline age, vertical and horizontal cup-disc ratio, pattern standard deviation, IOP, and, especially, central corneal thickness are useful parameters in stratifying risk in patients with OHTN. Individuals at high risk of developing POAG may benefit from more frequent examinations and early preventive treatment.

CLINICAL CASE: 60-YEAR-OLD WOMAN WITH OCULAR HYPERTENSION

Case History

A 60-year-old Caucasian woman presents for a routine examination after noticing that she is having trouble seeing up close. She denies any other ocular complaints. Her last eye exam was as a teenager. On examination, her visual acuity is 20/40 in the right eye and 20/30 in the left eye uncorrected, with J3 in both eyes at near. Manifest refraction reveals a +1.75 correction and a best corrected vision acuity of 20/30 in both eyes. She is found to have 1+ nuclear sclerotic cataract. Intraocular pressure is 24 mm Hg in both eyes and gonioscopy shows open angles. Dilated fundus examination reveals no abnormalities other than symmetrically enlarged cup-to-disc ratios of 0.5. Both optic discs respect the "ISNT" rule (normal eyes show a characteristic configuration for disc rim thickness of inferior ≥ superior ≥ nasal ≥ temporal).[7] Automated perimetry reveals no abnormalities (Humphrey pattern standard deviation mean = 1.8 dB) and optical coherence tomography of the nerve fiber layer does not show thinning. What additional testing or piece of information would be most helpful in determining the risk of developing glaucoma in this patient?

A. Family history of glaucoma.
B. Ishahara color plates.
C. Age.
D. Pachymetry for central corneal thickness.

Suggested Answer

The examination findings in this asymptomatic patient with moderately elevated IOP are relatively benign indicating that she would be classified as OHTN. Based on the OHTS and the pooled OHTS-EGPS predictive model,[8] the most important determinant for her risk of progression is central corneal thickness (option D). This woman's central corneal thickness was 490 μm, giving her an estimated 5-year risk of developing POAG in at least one eye of 20%, which is significant (https://ohts.wustl.edu/risk/). Based on this, she would likely warrant IOP-lowering therapy and frequent follow-up to detect progression to glaucomatous optic neuropathy.

References

1. Kass MA, Heuer DK, Higginbotham EJ, et al.. The Ocular Hypertension Treatment Study: a randomized trial determines that topical ocular hypotensive medication delays or prevents the onset of primary open-angle glaucoma. *Arch Ophthalmol.* 2002;120(6):701–13.
2. Gordon MO, Kass MA, for the Ocular Hypertension Treatment Study Group. The Ocular Hypertension Treatment Study: design and baseline description of the participants. *Arch Ophthalmol.* 1999;117573–83.
3. Singh K, Spaeth G, Zimmerman T, Minckler D. Target pressure—glaucomatologists' holey grail. *Ophthalmology.* 2000;107:629–30.
4. Higginbotham EJ, Gordon MO, Beiser JA, et al.; Ocular Hypertension Treatment Study Group. The Ocular Hypertension Treatment Study: topical medication delays or prevents primary open-angle glaucoma in African American individuals. *Arch Ophthalmol.* 2004;122(6):813–20.
5. Gordon MO, Beiser JA, Brandt JD, et al., for the Ocular Hypertension Treatment Study Group. The Ocular Hypertension Treatment Study: baseline factors that predict the onset of primary open-angle glaucoma. *Arch Ophthalmol.* 2002;120:714–20.
6. Kass MA, Gordon MO, Gao F, et al.; Ocular Hypertension Treatment Study Group. Delaying treatment of ocular hypertension: the ocular hypertension treatment study. *Arch Ophthalmol.* 2010;128(3):276–87.
7. Harizman N, Oliveira C, Chiang A, et al. The ISNT rule and differentiation of normal from glaucomatous eyes. *Arch Ophthalmol.* 2006;124(11):1579–83.
8. The Ocular Hypertension Treatment Study (OHTS) Group and the European Glaucoma Prevention Study (EGPS) Group. A validated prediction model for the development of primary open-angle glaucoma in individuals with ocular hypertension. *Ophthalmology.* 2007;114(1):10–19.

16

Intraocular Pressure Control and Long-Term Visual Field Loss in Open-Angle Glaucoma[*]

Collaborative Initial Glaucoma Treatment Study (CIGTS)

> These results support considering more aggressive treatment when undue elevation or variation in intraocular measures is observed.
> —MUSCH ET AL[1]

Research Question: Are patients with newly diagnosed open-angle glaucoma managed better by initial treatment with medications or by immediate filtration surgery?[1]

Funding: National Eye Institute, National Institutes of Health.

Year Study Began: 1993.

Year Study Published: 2011.

Study Location: 14 centers in the United States.

Who Was Studied: Patients, 25–75 years of age, with primary open-angle (91%), pseudoexfoliation, or pigmentary glaucoma in one or both eyes, defined as intraocular pressures (IOPs) of 20 mm Hg or higher with visual field defects

[*] Basic and Clinical Science Course, Section 10: *Glaucoma*. San Francisco: American Academy of Ophthalmology; 2018–2019: 81, 111, 187–188.

and an optic disc appearance consistent with glaucoma, and preserved visual acuity (20/40 or better, approximately). The visual field defects had to include at least 3 contiguous points on the total deviation probability plot at the 2% level with a positive Glaucoma Hemifield Test. Patients with IOPs higher than 27 mm Hg with optic disc damage consistent with glaucomatous damage did not require visual field defects to be present. (The 29 subjects (4.8%) with pseudoexfoliation glaucoma were excluded from analyses because these subjects were older and their IOP at baseline was substantially higher than that of the other 2 diagnostic groups.)

Who Was Excluded: Patients were excluded from the study if they had used IOP eye drops for longer than 2 weeks or if eye drops were used at any point in the 3 weeks before the initial visit. Patients were also excluded if they had significant visual field defects at baseline or had undergone prior ocular surgery; if they had comorbid ocular disease such as proliferative diabetic retinopathy, moderate-severe nonproliferative diabetic retinopathy, or visually significant cataract; or other ocular conditions that could confound IOP measurement, including chronic use of corticosteroids.

How Many Patients: 607.

Study Overview: The CIGTS was a prospective, randomized clinical trial (Figure 16.1).[1,2]

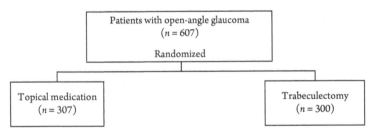

Figure 16.1. Summary of the CIGTS.

Study Intervention: Patients were randomized to either a stepped regimen of medications or initial trabeculectomy with or without 5-fluorouracil (5-FU). Patients in the medication arm started initially with a topical beta-blocker, then escalated to maximally tolerated topical medication +/- oral medication, if tolerated. If patients in either group did not meet their individualized target IOP (if the IOP was 1.0 mm Hg or more above target IOP) or had evidence of progressive visual field loss, defined as an increase in the visual field score of three units or more from the patient's reference visual field score, the next treatment step was argon laser trabeculoplasty (ALT).

Follow-Up: 3–9 years.

Endpoints: The primary outcome was progression of visual field defects, documented consistently over a 1-year period. Secondary outcomes included health-related quality of life, visual acuity and IOP.

RESULTS

- The mean IOP at baseline, before treatment initiation, was 27.6 mm Hg for medicine patients and 27.4 mm Hg for surgery patients. The mean IOP ranged from 17.1 to 18.3 in the medicine group and from 13.8 to 14.4 in the surgery group, based on all IOP measurements up to 3, 6, or 9 years.
  - The percentage of participants whose IOP was always <18 mm Hg decreased over time, ranging from 18% at 3 years to 8% at 9 years in the medicine group, and 59% at 3 years to 51% at 9 years in the surgery group.
- The mean deviation (MD) mean value on visual field testing at baseline was -5.2 dB in the medicine group and -5.7 dB in the surgery group. In the medicine group, MD mean values decreased from -5.1 dB at 3 years to -6.2 dB at 9 years. In the surgery group, MD mean values decreased from -5.3 dB at 3 years to -7.9 dB at 9 years.
  - The percentage of participants who had a -3-dB worsening from baseline increased from 11.5% to 17.4% to 23.1% in the medicine group, and from 9.4% to 10.9% to 34.1% in the surgery group, at 3, 6, and 9 years, respectively.
- After adjustment for baseline risk factors, in the medicine group larger values of 3 continuous IOP summary measures—maximum IOP ($P = .0003$), SD of IOP ($P = 0.0056$), and range of IOP ($P < .0001$)— were significantly associated with lower (worse) MD over the 3- to 9-year period. No IOP summary measure was significantly associated with MD over time in the surgery group.
  - The same 3 IOP summary measures were also significantly associated with substantial worsening of MD; however, the effects were similar in both treatment groups.

- For all but mean IOP, evidence of better IOP control (lower maximum IOP, less SD of IOP, and smaller range of IOP) was associated with a significantly beneficial effect in the medicine group, but no significant effect in the surgery group.
  - Those treated initially with medications whose maximum IOP was at the 75th percentile (24.0 mm Hg) had a pattern of MD decrease over time that was much more dramatic than that observed in medically-treated subjects whose maximum IOP was at the 25th percentile or that found in either surgery group.
- Three continuous IOP summary measures were significantly associated with substantial visual field loss. Interpreting these results for a 1 standard deviation (SD) increase in each summary measure shows that substantial visual field (VF) loss was associated with a larger range of IOP (odds ratio [OR] = 1.39), greater SD of IOP (OR = 1.37), and higher maximum IOP (OR = 1.34).
- No significant associations with substantial VF loss were found for any of the IOP threshold values (e.g., maintaining all IOP values below 16 or 18 mm Hg).
- Patients in the trabeculectomy arm required cataract surgery at a higher rate (17.3%) than those in the medical treatment arm (6.2%). The lower IOP rate in the surgery patients probably did not correlate with less visual field progression secondary to the development of cataracts.
- For the 3 measures of IOP variation during the follow-up that were identified as predictive for worse MD, the strongest predictive values were higher baseline IOP, black race, and a center effect.

Criticisms and Limitations: A total of 168 patients (27.7%) were enrolled with either moderate-to-severe visual field loss (despite being newly diagnosed) or no visual field loss. These participants may not have had glaucoma, but the authors argued that they would almost certainly have been treated outside of the study protocol.

Progression was judged solely on visual field change, which as more recent studies have shown, occurs later than structural progression as detected by optical coherence tomography.[3]

The role of factors now recognized to be important, such as IOP fluctuation, diurnal variation, and central corneal thickness, could not be assessed, as IOP and MD measurements were made at 6-monthly visits and information on central corneal thickness was available on a subset only.

Other Relevant Studies and Information:

- A U.S. Preventive Services Task Force (USPSTF) systematic review comparing the effectiveness of medical, laser, and surgical treatments in adults with open-angle glaucoma concluded that there was high-level evidence that medical treatment and trabeculectomy reduce the risk for optic nerve damage and visual field loss compared with no treatment, but that the comparative efficacy of different treatments was not clear.[4]
- Further analysis of data from the CIGTS found the percentage of participants showing substantial visual field improvement (defined as change from baseline of ≥ 3 decibels in MD) over time was similar to that showing VF loss through 5 years after initial treatment, after which VF loss became more frequent. Measures of better IOP control during treatment significantly predictive of VF improvement included a lower mean IOP, a lower minimum IOP, and lower sustained levels of IOP over follow-up.[5]

Summary and Implications: Three measures of IOP fluctuation over extended time, the range of IOP, the SD of IOP, and the maximum IOP, seem to play an important role in visual field progression, particularly among those treated medically. Monitoring for IOP fluctuation seems advisable, and more aggressive treatment should be considered when undue elevation or variation in IOP measures is observed.

CLINICAL CASE: AN ELDERLY MAN WITH POORLY CONTROLLED GLAUCOMA

Case History

A 65-year-old African American man with a past medical history of asthma, an allergy to sulfa, and a past ocular history of glaucoma and cataract surgery presents to your clinic for evaluation. From his history you learn that he has been followed for decades by a nonsurgical eye care provider who is now retired. The patient presents to you all of the handwritten notes from the past 10 years of visits with the now retired eye care provider. Review of the records reveals that he has been on topical brimonidine 0.2% and latanoprost 0.015% for years. His IOP measurements over the past 10 years have been recorded every 6 months and reveal a maximum IOP of 26 mm Hg and a range of IOP from 15 to 26 mm Hg, but with very few IOP readings below 18 mm Hg. There was no optical coherence tomography (OCT) report but the records did include three visual fields done in the past 5 years. These reveal worsening arcuate defects in both eyes. You obtain an OCT, which confirms your examination suspicion of glaucomatous damage to his optic nerves. The patient's IOP in your clinic is 21 mm Hg in both eyes. The visual field done in your clinic reveals a worse MD compared to the previous visual fields done by the retired provider. Based on results from CIGTS, your recommendation for this patient would most likely be which of the following?

A. Add pilocarpine because there is pigment on gonioscopy and the CIGTS recommends maximum medical therapy in pigmentary glaucoma patients before proceeding to surgery.

B. Send the patient to an allergist for sulfa allergy testing and, if it is negative, add a topical and/or oral carbonic anhydrase inhibitor because the CIGTS recommends maximum medical therapy in pigmentary glaucoma patients before proceeding to surgery.

C. Observe the patient's IOP range and the MD on his visual field testing over the next couple of years to ensure the worsening MD meets criteria according to CIGTS to justify the risk of surgery.

D. Based on your review of records which reveals the patient's range and maximum IOPs on medical treatment, send the patient for glaucoma surgery evaluation since, based on the findings of the CIGTS, he is at high risk for continued visual field progression.

Suggested Answer
Option D.

References

1. Musch DC, Gillespie BW, Niziol LM, Lichter PR, Varma R; CIGTS Study Group. Intraocular pressure control and long-term visual field loss in the Collaborative Initial Glaucoma Treatment Study. *Ophthalmology.* 2011;118(9):1766–73.

2. Musch DC, Lichter PR, Guire KE, Standardi CL. The Collaborative Initial Glaucoma Treatment Study: study design, methods, and baseline characteristics of enrolled patients. *Ophthalmology.* 1999;106(4):653–62.

3. Wishart PK. Interpretation of the glaucoma "landmark studies." *Br J Ophthalmol.* 2009;93(5):561–2.

4. Boland MV, Ervin AM, Friedman DS, et al. Comparative effectiveness of treatments for open-angle glaucoma: a systematic review for the U.S. Preventive Services Task Force. *Ann Intern Med.* 2013;158(4):271–9.

5. Musch DC, Gillespie BW, Palmberg PF, Spaeth G, Niziol LM, Lichter PR. Visual field improvement in the collaborative initial glaucoma treatment study. *Am J Ophthalmol.* 2014;158(1):96–104.e2.

17

Latanoprost for Open-Angle Glaucoma[*]

United Kingdom Glaucoma Treatment Study (UKGTS)

This is the first randomized placebo-controlled trial to show preservation of the visual field with an intraocular-pressure-lowering drug in patients with open-angle glaucoma.

—GARWAY-HEATH ET AL[1]

Research Question: Does latanoprost, a prostaglandin analogue, preserve visual field longer than placebo?[1]

Funding: Pfizer; UK National Institute for Health Research Biomedical Research Center.

Year Study Began: 2006.

Year Study Published: 2015.

Study Location: 10 centers in the United Kingdom.

Who Was Studied: Patients with newly diagnosed, untreated open-angle glaucoma, defined as the presence of glaucomatous visual field defects in at least one eye with corresponding damage to the optic nerve head and an open iridocorneal

[*] Basic and Clinical Science Course, Section 10. *Glaucoma*. San Francisco: American Academy of Ophthalmology, 2018–2019.

drainage angle on gonioscopy. Patients with pseudoexfoliation glaucoma were eligible.

Who Was Excluded: Patients with pigment dispersion glaucoma were excluded. Other exclusion criteria included advanced glaucoma (visual field mean deviation worse than −10 dB in the better eye or −16 dB in the worse eye), mean baseline intraocular pressure (IOP) of 30 mm Hg or higher, Snellen visual acuity worse than 20/40 (6/12), and poor image quality (>40 μm mean pixel height standard deviation) with the Heidelberg retina tomograph (Heidelberg Engineering, Heidelberg, Germany).

How Many Patients: 516.

Study Overview: This was a randomized, triple-masked, placebo-controlled trial (Figure 17.1).[1-3]

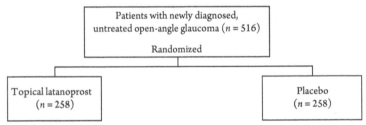

Figure 17.1. Summary of the UKGTS.

Study Intervention: Participants were randomly allocated to receive either latanoprost 0.005% or latanoprost vehicle eye drops (placebo) alone once a day in both eyes.

Follow-Up: 24 months.

Endpoints: The primary measure of outcome was time to visual field deterioration within 24 months. Specifically, visual field deterioration was defined as at least three visual field locations worse than baseline at the 5% levels in two consecutive reliable visual fields and at least three visual field locations worse than baseline at the 5% levels in the two subsequent consecutive reliable visual fields. Additional endpoints were IOP higher than 35 mm Hg on two successive occasions and visual acuity reduction to less than 20/60 (6/18).

RESULTS

- 59 of (25.6%) 230 patients in the placebo group showed visual field deterioration consistent with glaucomatous progression by 24 months compared with 35 (15.2%) of 231 in the latanoprost group (P= .006)
  - Of the 94 patients with visual field deterioration, time to first deterioration was significantly longer in the latanoprost group than in the placebo group (adjusted hazard ratio[HR] 0.44; P= .0003)
    - In participants reaching a visual field endpoint, the mean change in mean deviation was −1.6 dB.
  - Treatment differences were evident at 18 months (HR 0.43; P = .001) and 12 months (HR 0.47; P= .035)
- At 24 months the mean IOP reduction from baseline (after adjustment for missing data) was 3.8 mm Hg in the latanoprost group and 0.9 mm Hg in the placebo group.
- 18 serious adverse events were reported (9 in each group); none were attributed to the study drug.

Criticisms and Limitations: A potential limitation of the UKGTS was the relatively high loss to (or incomplete) follow-up, which could reduce the generalizability of the results. However, individuals lost to follow-up were generally similar to those remaining in the trial. In addition, participant ascertainment was not population-based, but based on referral from primary care (community optometry practice). The UKGTS participants were predominantly white (about 90%), which might also reduce generalizability of the findings to other populations that might exhibit greater susceptibility to vision loss. Furthermore, individuals with advanced open-angle glaucoma were excluded so that the results of the trial only apply to patients with mild to moderate glaucoma.

Other Relevant Studies and Information:

- A small prospective study of the effects of topical pranoprofen, a nonsteroidal anti-inflammatory drug on IOP and the ocular surface in primary open-angle glaucoma patients treated with topical latanoprost 0.005% showed that the combination of pranoprofen can not only significantly enhance the latanoprost-induced IOP-lowering effect but also relieve the uncomfortable ocular symptoms caused by latanoprost.[4]

Summary and Implications: The UKGTS was the first placebo-controlled trial to show visual field preservation through lowering of intraocular pressure with topical drugs in patients with open-angle glaucoma, and the first to show the visual-field-preserving effect of a topical prostaglandin analogue.

Because two-thirds of patients in the placebo group had no detectable deterioration within 24 months, and the small amount of change needed for an endpoint occurred in just one eye of almost 90% of participants with data, the question arises as to whether some patients with glaucoma, particularly those with less visual field loss at baseline and those at lower risk of progression, could be monitored without treatment for a period. Investigators have previously suggested initial careful observation without treatment in patients with open-angle glaucoma and normal tension glaucoma. Because deterioration patterns are difficult to predict, an observation period would be advantageous to identify patients who might not need treatment, thereby avoiding the unnecessary burden of treatment for such patients. The rate of progression of visual field loss might change over extended observation periods, and so regular reassessments of the rate of progression would be advisable.

CLINICAL CASE: A MIDDLE-AGED WOMAN WITH EARLY GLAUCOMA

Case History
A 62-year-old Caucasian woman presents for a routine eye exam and is found to have a glaucomatous visual field defect in one eye, with exam findings suspicious for corresponding damage to the optic nerve head, an open angle on gonioscopy, and an IOP of 27 mm Hg in both eyes. You discuss options with the patient and specifically refer to the UKGTS study. With regard to this study, which of the following is true?

A. It was the first glaucoma trial to compare a specific topical treatment to no treatment in patients with primary open-angle glaucoma.
B. It was the first placebo-controlled study to show visual field preservation using a topical drug (prostaglandin analog) in patients with primary open-angle glaucoma
C. It was the first study to consider visual field progression as a primary measure of outcome in patients with primary open-angle glaucoma

D. It was the first glaucoma study to compare results of surgical therapy with a prostaglandin analogue treatment in patients with primary open-angle glaucoma.

Suggested Answer
Option B.

References

1. Garway-Heath DF, Crabb DP, Bunce C, et al. Latanoprost for open-angle glaucoma (UKGTS): a randomised, multicentre, placebo-controlled trial. *Lancet.* 2015;385(9975):1295–304.
2. Garway-Heath DF, Lascaratos G, Bunce C, Crabb DP, Russell RA, Shah A. The United Kingdom Glaucoma Treatment Study: a multicenter, randomized, placebo-controlled clinical trial: design and methodology. *Ophthalmology.* 2013;120:68–76.
3. Lascaratos G, Garway-Heath DF, Burton R, et al. The United Kingdom Glaucoma Treatment Study: a multicenter, randomized, double-masked, placebo-controlled trial: baseline characteristics. *Ophthalmology.* 2013;120:2540–45.
4. Zhu S, Wang D, Han J. Effect of a topical combination of latanoprost and pranoprofen on intraocular pressure and the ocular surface in open-angle glaucoma patients. *J Ophthalmol.* 2018;2018:7474086.

18

Tube Shunt Surgery Versus Trabeculectomy in Eyes with Prior Ocular Surgery and Uncontrolled Glaucoma[*]

Tube Versus Trabeculectomy (TVT) Study

> The TVT Study does not demonstrate clear superiority of one glaucoma operation over the other, but indicates that both tube shunt surgery and trabeculectomy with mitomycin C are viable surgical options for treating medically uncontrolled glaucoma in patients with previous cataract extraction or failed filtering surgery.
>
> —GEDDE ET AL[1]

Research Question: Which has greater safety and efficacy in patients with uncontrolled glaucoma who have previously undergone cataract extraction with intraocular lens implantation and/or failed filtering surgery: tube shunt or trabeculectomy with mitomycin C (MMC)?[1]

Funding: Pfizer, Inc., New York, NY; Abbott Medical Optics, Santa Ana, CA; National Eye Institute, National Institutes of Health; Research to Prevent Blindness, Inc., New York, NY.

Year Study Began: 1999.

[*] Basic and Clinical Science Course, Section 10. *Glaucoma*. San Francisco: American Academy of Ophthalmology; 2018–2019: 215–217.

Year Study Published: 2012.

Study Location: 17 centers in the United States and the United Kingdom.

Who Was Studied: Patients, 18 to 85 years old, with previous trabeculectomy and/or cataract extraction with intraocular lens implantation, and intraocular pressure (IOP) ≥ 18 mm Hg and ≤ 40 mm Hg on maximum tolerated medical therapy.

Who Was Excluded: Patients were excluded if they had no light perception, active iris neovascularization or proliferative retinopathy, iridocorneal endo-thelial syndrome, epithelial or fibrous downgrowth, aphakia, vitreous in the anterior chamber for which a vitrectomy was anticipated, chronic or recurrent uveitis, severe posterior blepharitis, unwillingness to discontinue contact lens use after surgery, previous cyclodestructive procedure, prior scleral buckling procedure, presence of silicone oil, conjunctival scarring precluding a superior trabeculectomy, or a need for glaucoma surgery combined with other ocular procedures or anticipated need for additional ocular surgery.

How Many Patients: 212.

Study Overview: The TVT was a randomized clinical trial (Figure 18.1).[1,2]

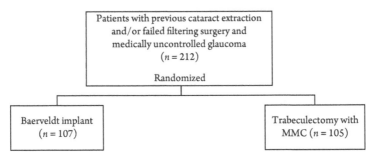

Figure 18.1. Summary of the TVT study.

Study Intervention: The patients were randomly allocated to receive either a 350-mm² Baerveldt glaucoma implant or a trabeculectomy with MMC. Only 1 eye of each eligible patient was included in the study.

Follow-Up: 5 years.

Endpoints: IOP, visual acuity (VA), use of supplemental medical therapy, surgical complications, visual fields, quality of life, and failure. Failure was defined as IOP > 21 mm Hg or less than 20% reduction below baseline on 2 consecutive follow-up visits for 3 months, IOP ≤ 5 mm Hg on 2 consecutive follow-up visits after 3 months, reoperation for glaucoma, or loss of light perception vision. Reoperation for glaucoma was defined as additional glaucoma surgery requiring a return to the operating room, such as placement of a tube shunt. Cyclodestruction was also counted as a reoperation for glaucoma. Eyes that did not fail and were not on supplemental medical therapy were defined as a complete success; eyes that had not failed but required supplemental medical therapy were defined as qualified successes.

RESULTS

- At 5 years, IOP was 14.4 ± 6.9 mm Hg in the tube group and 12.6 ± 5.9 in the trabeculectomy group ($P = .12$).
- At 5 years, IOP reduction from baseline was 10.2 ± 7.4 mm Hg (41.4%) in the tube group ($P < .001$) and 12.4 ± 7.2 mm Hg (49.5%) in the trabeculectomy group ($P < .001$).
  - IOP reduction was similar between the two groups at 5 years ($P = .097$).
  - The proportion of patients with IOP ≤14 mm Hg was also similar between the tube (63.9%) and trabeculectomy (63.5%) groups ($P > .99$).
- Use of glaucoma medications was reduced in both groups from baseline, 1.8 ± 1.8 in the tube group ($P < .001$) and 1.7 ± 2.0 in the trabeculectomy group ($P < .001$) after completing 5 year follow-up.
  - There was a significantly greater use of medication in the tube group compared to the trabeculectomy group in the first 2 postop years, but the mean number of medications was similar at year 3 and after.
- There was a significantly higher failure rate in the trabeculectomy group as opposed to the tube group after 5 years. Failure occurred in 24 (33%) of patients in the tube group and 42 (50%) of patients in the trabeculectomy group ($P = .034$).
  - Cumulative probability of failure was 29.8% in the tube group and 46.9% in the trabeculectomy group at 5 years ($P = .002$).
- In the tube group, 18 (21%) patients were a complete success and 31 (42%) patients were qualified successes; in the trabeculectomy group, 24 (29%) were a complete success and 18 (21%) patients were qualified successes.

- While the tube group had a higher overall success rate after 5 years, the rate of complete success was similar between treatment groups ($P = .58$).
- A higher reoperation rate was seen in the trabeculectomy group (29%) versus the tube group (9%) ($P = .025$).
- Significant vision loss was noted in both groups over the 5-year follow-up period, but the difference was not statistically significant.
  - In the tube group, logMAR Snellen VA decreased .38 ± .72 units from baseline ($P < .001$) and Early Treatment Diabetic Retinopathy Study (ETDRS). VA was decreased by 15 ± 26 letters from baseline ($P = .001$); in the trabeculectomy group, logMAR Snellen VA decreased .34 ± .60 units ($P < .001$) and ETDRS VA decreased 14 ± 25 letters ($P = .001$).
  - The rate of loss of 2 or more lines of Snellen VA was similar between the tube (46%) and trabeculectomy (43%) groups at 5 years ($P = .93$).

Criticisms and Limitations: The study results cannot be generalized to other patient groups, such as neovascular glaucoma, which are more resistant to treatment. Nor can the results be applied to other implant types. Furthermore, although much of the surgical procedure was standardized, some variation in surgical technique was permitted.

At the time of the study, higher dosages of MMC were used than are used presently. This could possibly be associated with higher rates of hypotony and lower rate of bleb fibrosis.

Clinicians were not masked to the treatment assignment of patients, which could introduce a bias in their judgment about when to reoperate. However, the study did evaluate the mean IOP at time of failure and reoperation and found no significant difference between the two groups so it appears that no selection bias was present.

Other Relevant Studies and Information:

- A meta-analysis of 6 clinical trials comparing Ahmed glaucoma valve (AGV) implantation with trabeculectomy concluded that AGV was equivalent to trabeculectomy in reducing the IOP, the number of glaucoma medications, success rates, and rates of the most common complications, but that AGV was associated with a significantly lower frequency of overall adverse events.[3]

- A Cochrane review of the effectiveness and safety of aqueous shunts in general concluded: "Information was insufficient to conclude whether there are differences between aqueous shunts and trabeculectomy for glaucoma treatment. While the Baerveldt implant may lower IOP more than the Ahmed implant, the evidence was of moderate-certainty and it is unclear whether the difference in IOP reduction is clinically significant. Overall, methodology and data quality among existing randomized controlled trials of aqueous shunts was heterogeneous across studies, and there are no well-justified or widely accepted generalizations about the superiority of one surgical procedure or device over another."[4]

Summary and Implications: Both tube shunt surgery and trabeculectomy with MMC are viable surgical options for treating medically uncontrolled glaucoma in patients with previous cataract extraction or failed filtering surgery. There is no clear superiority of one glaucoma operation over the other, although the tube shunt had a higher success rate in comparison to the trabeculectomy with MMC over 5 years of follow-up. Both procedures had similar IOP reduction and similar use of supplemental medications. The rate of reoperation was higher in the group undergoing trabeculectomy with MMC than in the tube shunt group. Vision loss was noted to occur at a similar rate in both groups.

CLINICAL CASE: A YOUNG WOMAN WITH PREVIOUS CATARACT SURGERY AND UNCONTROLLED GLAUCOMA

Case History

A 43-year-old African American woman comes to your clinic to establish care. She has a history of cataract extraction and intraocular lens implant for traumatic cataract in the right eye and juvenile glaucoma. She is currently on combination timolol/dorzolamide drops twice daily, brimonidine three times daily, and travoprost nightly. Her VA is 20/30 in the right eye and 20/20 in the left eye, IOP is 20 mm Hg in the right eye and 14 mm Hg in the left eye. On fundus exam, both optic discs are without edema or pallor, the cup-to-disc ratio is 0.8 in the right eye and 0.6 in the left eye, and the anterior chamber angles are open to the scleral spur 360° in both eyes. Optical coherence tomography shows superior thinning of the retinal nerve fiber layer in the right eye but is normal in the left eye. Visual field examination shows progression of an inferior arcuate defect in the right eye compared to her records from her previous provider. Based on these findings, what would be the recommended treatment for this patient according to the TVT study?

A. Baerveldt tube shunt and trabeculectomy both lower IOP effectively. The trabeculectomy typically lowers the IOP slightly more, but the tube shunt has a lower rate of failure after 5 years.
B. Baerveldt tube shunt and trabeculectomy are equal in every way, and the decision is typically up to physician preference.
C. Baerveldt tube shunt and trabeculectomy both lower IOP effectively. The tube shunt typically lowers the IOP slightly more and has a lower rate of failure after 5 years.
D. Baerveldt tube shunt and trabeculectomy both lower IOP effectively. The trabeculectomy typically lowers the IOP slightly more and has a lower rate of failure after 5 years.

Suggested Answer

Option A. According to the TVT study, the trabeculectomy group had a slightly lower (though not statistically significant) IOP after 5 years. However, the patients in the tube shunt group had a lower failure rate than the trabeculectomy group at 5 years.

References

1. Gedde SJ, Schiffman JC, Feuer WJ, Herndon LW, Brandt JD, Budenz DL; Tube versus Trabeculectomy Study Group. Treatment outcomes in the Tube Versus Trabeculectomy (TVT) study after five years of follow-up. *Am J Ophthalmol.* 2012;153(5):789–803.
2. Gedde SJ, Schiffman JC, Feuer WJ, Parrish RK 2nd, Heuer DK, Brandt JD; Tube Versus Trabeculectomy Study Group. The Tube Versus Trabeculectomy Study: design and baseline characteristics of study patients. *Am J Ophthalmol.* 2005;140(2):275–87.
3. HaiBo T, Xin K, ShiHeng L, Lin L. Comparison of Ahmed glaucoma valve implantation and trabeculectomy for glaucoma: a systematic review and meta-analysis. *PLoS One.* 2015;10(2):e0118142.
4. Tseng VL, Coleman AL, Chang MY, Caprioli J. Aqueous shunts for glaucoma. *Cochrane Database Syst Rev.* 2017;7:CD004918.

19

Pooled Data Analysis of the Ahmed Baerveldt Comparison Study and the Ahmed Versus Baerveldt Study[*]

Ahmed Baerveldt Comparison (ABC) Study, Ahmed Versus Baerveldt (AVB) Study

The Baerveldt group had a lower failure rate, lower rate of *de novo* glaucoma surgery, and lower mean IOP on fewer medications than the Ahmed group. Baerveldt implantation carried a higher risk of hypotony.

—CHRISTAKIS ET AL[1]

Research Question: Is the Ahmed-FP7 or the Baerveldt BG101-350 implant more efficacious in the treatment of refractory or high-risk glaucoma?[1]

Funding: The ABC study was funded by the National Eye Institute, National Institutes of Health; New World Medical, Inc. (Rancho Cucamonga, CA); Abbott Medical Optics (Abbott Park, IL); Glaucoma Research Society of Canada (Toronto, Canada); and Research to Prevent Blindness (New York, NY). The AVB study was funded by the Glaucoma Research Society of Canada (Toronto, Canada) and Research to Prevent Blindness (New York, NY).

Year Study Began: ABC—2006; AVB—2005.

[*] Basic and Clinical Science Course, Section 10. *Glaucoma*. San Francisco: American Academy of Ophthalmology; 2018–2019: 214.

Year Study Published: 2017.

Study Location: 22 centers in the United States, Canada, the United Kingdom, Chile, Singapore, and Brazil.

Who Was Studied: Eligibility criteria were the same in the 2 studies: (1) 18 years or older; (2) uncontrolled glaucoma, defined as IOP greater than clinical target despite maximum tolerated medical therapy; (3) patients who had previously failed trabeculectomy were included; (4) high-risk glaucoma, including neovascular and uveitic glaucoma, were included.

Who Was Excluded: The following were the exclusion criteria for both studies: (1) scheduled to undergo an additional procedure at the time of device implantation (e.g., cataract surgery, corneal transplant); (2) prior cyclodestructive procedure; (3) no light perception vision. Additionally, the ABC study excluded patients who had uveitis secondary to a systemic condition (e.g., juvenile rheumatoid arthritis), patients with glaucoma associated with elevated episcleral venous pressure, and patients who had silicone oil in the operative eye.

How Many Patients: 514 patients (ABC—276; AVB—238). Only 1 eye per patient was eligible for enrollment.

Study Overview: The ABC and AVB studies were independent randomized clinical trials.[2,3] The study design, patient population, and outcome criteria were similar, allowing the data to be pooled.[4,5] The data were recategorized using a common methodology to address data heterogeneity.

Study Intervention: Patients were randomized to receive either an Ahmed valve (Model AGV FP7) implant or a Baerveldt implant (Model 101-350 BGI) by an experienced surgeon using standardized techniques. Both studies were open-label trials, so both the surgeon and the patient were aware of the treatment arm.

Follow-Up: 5 years.

Endpoints: The primary outcome criteria for both studies was failure, defined as (1) IOP > 18 mm Hg or IOP < 6 mm Hg or IOP reduced less than 20% from baseline, for 2 consecutive visits after 3 months; (2) de novo glaucoma procedure (e.g., cyclodestruction, additional tube shunt); (3) loss of light perception or severe vision loss; or (4) removal of the implant.

RESULTS

- The mean IOP in the Ahmed group decreased from 31.2 ± 10.9 mm Hg preoperatively to 15.8 ± 5.2 mm Hg at 5 years (49% reduction, $P < .001$). The mean IOP in the Baerveldt group decreased from 31.8 ± 11.8 mm Hg preoperatively to 13.2 ± 4.8 mm Hg at 5 years.
  - The Baerveldt group had a lower mean IOP at all postop visits beginning at 6 months and continuing through 5 years ($P < .05$).
- Both devices reduced the need for glaucoma medications. The mean number of medications used in the Ahmed group decreased from 3.3 ± 1.1 preoperatively to 1.9 ± 1.5 at 5 years (42% reduction, $P < .001$). The mean number of glaucoma medications used in the Baerveldt group decreased from 3.3 ± 1.1 preoperatively to 1.5 ± 1.4 at 5 years (55% reduction, $P < .001$).
  - The Baerveldt group required fewer glaucoma medications at all postop appointments beginning at 6 months and continuing through 5 years ($P < .05$).
- At 5 years, the cumulative proportion of failing was 49% in the Ahmed group and 37% in the Baerveldt group ($P = .01$). The relative hazard of treatment failure in the Ahmed group was 1.34 times that of the Baerveldt group ($P = .03$).
  - The most common reason for failure was high IOP in both groups, which accounted for 112 (42%) of the failures in the Ahmed group and 56 (23%) of the failures in the Baerveldt group.
  - Failure due to hypotony occurred in 0.4% of the Ahmed group and 4.5% of the Baerveldt group ($P = .002$).
- Visual outcomes were similar between groups ($P = .90$).
  - Mean logMAR acuity in the Ahmed group worsened from 1.2 ± 1.0 preoperatively to 1.5 ± 1.2 at 5 years ($P < .001$). Mean logMAR acuity in the Baerveldt group worsened from 1.1 ± 1.0 preoperatively to 1.5 ± 1.3 at 5 years. Both groups had similar visual acuities at all postop appointments ($P > .05$).
  - Severe vision loss occurred in 13 (5%) patients in the Ahmed group and 18 (7%) patients in the Baerveldt group ($P = .27$).
- The cumulative proportion of patients requiring de novo glaucoma surgery was 17% in the Ahmed group and 9% in the Baerveldt group ($P = .01$). The relative risk of requiring de novo surgery in the Ahmed group was 2 times higher than that of the Baerveldt group ($P = .010$).
- Device explantation was required in 4 (2%) patients in the Ahmed group and 6 (2%) patients in the Baerveldt group ($P = .002$).

Criticisms and Limitations: The study population had advanced glaucoma with significant visual deficits that limited reliability of the visual field tests that guided treatment decisions and might have resulted in insufficient power to detect small changes in vision between the two groups.

These patients had high rates of secondary glaucoma that failed previous trabeculectomy with antimetabolite. As such, the results may not be as applicable to patients who are having shunt placement as an initial surgical intervention.

The surgeon was not masked to what treatment arm the patient was in, which could allow biases in postop clinical management (e.g., when to start patient on medications or to perform de novo glaucoma surgery).

A population-based IOP target (6–18 mm Hg) was used as an objective, standardized way to compare the groups, but it may not reflect the true treatment goal of individual patients based on their preoperative IOP, glaucoma subtype and severity, and threshold for progression.

Other Relevant Studies and Information:

- A study of the long-term surgical outcomes of the Baerveldt 250 mm^2 versus Baerveldt 350 mm^2 glaucoma drainage implants (GDIs) in the treatment of refractory glaucoma showed that, with a mean follow-up of 40 and 31 months, no differences in surgical success, VA, IOP, number of medications at the last visit, and complication/failure rates were noted between the Baerveldt 250 mm^2 versus Baerveldt 350 mm^2 GDIs, respectively. The size of the GDI may not be associated with surgical outcomes.[6]
- A meta-analysis of 6 studies comparing the Ahmed glaucoma valve (AGV) implant and the Baerveldt implant for the treatment of refractory glaucoma concluded: "The Baerveldt implant is more effective in both its surgical success rate and reducing glaucoma medication, but it is comparable to the AGV implant in lowering IOP. Both implants may have comparable incidences of adverse events."[7]
- A Cochrane review of the effectiveness and safety of aqueous shunts in general concluded: "Information was insufficient to conclude whether there are differences between aqueous shunts and trabeculectomy for glaucoma treatment. While the Baerveldt implant may lower IOP more than the Ahmed implant, the evidence was of moderate-certainty and it is unclear whether the difference in IOP reduction is clinically significant. Overall, methodology and data quality among existing randomized controlled trials of aqueous shunts was heterogeneous across studies, and there are no well-justified or widely accepted

generalizations about the superiority of one surgical procedure or device over another."[8]

- For recent reviews of glaucoma drainage implants, see [9] and [10].

Summary and Implications: Both devices lowered IOP and the need for glaucoma medications. The Baerveldt implant had lower failure rates, lower rates of *de novo* glaucoma surgery, and patients had lower IOP on fewer medications at the 5-year end of the studies in comparison to the Ahmed implants, but had a higher risk for hypotony. The selection of a device for a patient should be based on target IOP, compliance with medications, urgency for IOP lowering, surgeon familiarity with each device, and the surgeon's personal outcomes with the individual devices.

CLINICAL CASE: AN ELDERLY WOMAN WITH UNCONTROLLED GLAUCOMA DESPITE MEDICAL TREATMENT

Case History

An 82-year-old African American woman is brought to your clinic by her daughter for follow-up for open-angle glaucoma and a new glasses prescription. The patient is currently on timolol/dorzolamide combination BID and latanoprost. Her daughter informs you that her mother was recently diagnosed with dementia and frequently misses doses of her medication during the week due to poor memory. Her corrected VA is 20/25 in the right eye and 20/30 in the left eye and her applanated IOP is 19 mm Hg in the right eye and 23 mm Hg in the left eye. Optical coherence tomography at this visit shows progressive thinning of the retinal nerve fiber layer in the left eye. The patient is refracted, and her prescription is $-7.00 + 0.25 \times 168$ (right) and $-7.25 + 0.25 \times 004$ (left). Her daughter asks what would be the best next step to stop further damage to her left eye. What would be your recommendation according to the pooled data from the ABC and AVB studies?

A. Ahmed tube shunts are more effective at lowering IOP and have a lower risk of hypotony than Baerveldt tube shunts.
B. Ahmed tube shunts are less effective at lowering IOP but have a lower risk of hypotony than Baerveldt tube shunts.
C. Ahmed tube shunts and Baerveldt tube shunts are equally effective in lowering IOP and in their risk of hypotony.

> D. Ahmed tube shunts are less effective at lowering IOP and have a lower risk of hypotony than Baerveldt tube shunts.
>
> **Suggested Answer**
> Option B. According to the pooled data of the ABC and AVB studies, the Ahmed tube shunt had lower rates of hypotony as opposed to Baerveldt shunts but were not quite as effective at lowering IOP.

References

1. Christakis PG, Zhang D, Budenz DL, Barton K, Tsai JC, Ahmed IIK; ABC-AVB Study Groups. Five-year pooled data analysis of the Ahmed Baerveldt Comparison study and the Ahmed Versus Baerveldt study. *Am J Ophthalmol.* 2017;176:118–26.
2. Barton K, Gedde SJ, Budenz DL, Feuer WJ, Schiffman J; Ahmed Baerveldt Comparison Study Group. The Ahmed Baerveldt Comparison Study methodology, baseline patient characteristics, and intraoperative complications. *Ophthalmology.* 2011;118(3):435–42.
3. Christakis PG, Tsai JC, Zurakowski D, Kalenak JW, Cantor LB, Ahmed II. The Ahmed Versus Baerveldt study: design, baseline patient characteristics, and intraoperative complications. *Ophthalmology.* 2011;118(11):2172–9.
4. Budenz DL, Barton K, Gedde SJ, Feuer WJ, Schiffman J, Costa VP, Godfrey DG, Buys YM; Ahmed Baerveldt Comparison Study Group. Five-year treatment outcomes in the Ahmed Baerveldt comparison study. *Ophthalmology.* 2015;122(2):308–16.
5. Christakis PG, Kalenak JW, Tsai JC, Zurakowski D, Kammer JA, Harasymowycz PJ, Mura JJ, Cantor LB, Ahmed II. The Ahmed Versus Baerveldt Study: five-year treatment outcomes. *Ophthalmology.* 2016;123(10):2093–102.
6. Allan EJ, Khaimi MA, Jones JM, Ding K, Skuta GL. Long-term efficacy of the Baerveldt 250 mm² compared with the Baerveldt 350 mm² implant. *Ophthalmology.* 2015;122(3):486–93.
7. Wang S, Gao X, Qian N. The Ahmed shunt versus the Baerveldt shunt for refractory glaucoma: a meta-analysis. *BMC Ophthalmol.* 2016;16:83.
8. Tseng VL, Coleman AL, Chang MY, Caprioli J. Aqueous shunts for glaucoma. *Cochrane Database Syst Rev.* 2017;7:CD004918.
9. Ashburn FS, Netland PA. The evolution of glaucoma drainage implants. *J Ophthalmic Vis Res.* 2018;13(4):498–500.
10. Chen J, Gedde SJ. New developments in tube shunt surgery. *Curr Opin Ophthalmol.* 2019;30(2):125–31.

20

Risk Factors for Branch and Central Retinal Vein Occlusion*

The Eye Disease Case-Control Study

An increased risk of branch retinal vein occlusion was found in persons with a history of systemic hypertension, cardiovascular disease, increased BMI at 20 years of age, a history of glaucoma, and higher serum levels of alpha 2 globulin. Risk was decreased with higher levels of alcohol consumption and high density lipoprotein cholesterol.

—EYE DISEASE CASE-CONTROL STUDY GROUP[1]

An increased risk of central retinal vein occlusion was found in persons with systemic hypertension, diabetes mellitus, and open-angle glaucoma. Risk of CRVO decreased with increasing levels of physical activity and increasing levels of alcohol consumption. In women, risk of occlusion decreased with use of postmenopausal estrogens but increased with higher erythrocyte sedimentation rates (ESR).

—EYE DISEASE CASE-CONTROL STUDY GROUP[2]

Research Question: What are the risk factors associated with developing a branch retinal vein occlusion (BRVO) or a central retinal vein occlusion (CRVO)?[1,2]

---

* Basic and Clinical Science Course, Section 12. *Retina and Vitreous*. San Francisco: American Academy of Ophthalmology; 2018–2019: 125–128.

Funding: National Eye Institute, National Institutes of Health.

Year Study Began: 1986.

Year Study Published: 1993 (BRVO) and 1996 (CRVO).

Study Location: 5 clinical centers in the United States.

Who Was Studied: Patients between the ages of 21and 80 years of age with BRVO or CRVO, diagnosed in the year prior to enrollment. Cases of BRVO were required to have either flame-shaped or dot hemorrhages in the distribution of the occluded branch retinal vein with the apex located at an AV crossing; criteria were later expanded to include cases in which the retinal hemorrhages had resolved and new/collateral vessels had developed. Cases of CRVO were required to have flame-shaped, dot or punctate retinal hemorrhages or both in all four quadrants of the retina, dilation and increased tortuosity of the retinal veins, and optic disc swelling.

Who Was Excluded: Persons with other diseases included in the Eye Disease Case-Control Study (neovascular age-related macular degeneration [AMD], macular hole, retinal detachment), pathologic myopia, vasoproliferative retinopathy, intermediate or posterior intraocular inflammatory disease.

How Many Patients: 270 cases and 1,142 controls in the BRVO study; 258 cases (84 ischemic and 148 nonischemic) and 1,142 controls in the CRVO study (ischemic was defined as having at least 10 disc areas of nonperfusion on fluorescein angiography (FA)).

Study Overview: The Eye Disease Case-Control Study was a clinic-based, case-control study that investigated risk factors for 5 retinal diseases (BRVO, CRVO, neovascular AMD, idiopathic macular hole, and rhegmatogenous retinal detachment, using a similar protocol and the same large pool of controls.[1,2]

Study Intervention: None—this was a case-control study. Cases and controls were frequency matched for age, sex, and race.

Follow-Up: None—this was a case-control study.

Endpoints: Data on possible sociodemographic, clinical, ocular, and biochemical risk factors were collected using interview, eye and physical exam, and analysis of blood specimens.

RESULTS

BRVO:

- Patients had an increased risk of BRVO if they had a higher body mass index (BMI), history of diabetes or higher blood glucose levels, history of cardiovascular disease (CVD), higher levels of systolic or diastolic blood pressure (BP) or a history of hypertension, EKG irregularities, a history of glaucoma, higher IOP, increased alpha 2 globulin, and elevated triglycerides.
- Hypertension was found to be a particularly important risk factor for developing a BRVO.
  - Assuming the study sample is representative of the general population, then over 50% of BRVO cases can be attributed to hypertension.
  - Higher levels of HDL cholesterol, light to moderate alcohol consumption, and increased physical activity were associated with reduced risk of BRVO.

CRVO:

- Increased risk of CRVO was associated with history of diabetes mellitus and/or current treatment of diabetes, EKG irregularities, higher systolic and diastolic BP or hypertension, history of CVD, IOP in the contralateral eye, history of glaucoma, higher antithrombin III levels, and (in women) elevated ESR.
  - CVD, EKG irregularities, lower albumin-globulin ratio, higher alpha 1 globulin, higher blood glucose levels, and history of treatment for diabetes were associated with increased risk of ischemic CRVO only.
  - Systolic BP, diastolic BP, and hypertension were associated with both ischemic and nonischemic CRVO, but the odds ratio was higher for the ischemic subtype.
- Decreased risk of CRVO was associated with current mild to moderate alcohol consumption, amount of alcohol consumed daily (>1 oz vs. < 1 oz), education level, current or past physical activity, and (in postmenopausal women) with estrogen use (Table 20.1).

Table 20.1. ODDS RATIOS FOR RISK FACTORS ASSOCIATED WITH
BRVO AND CRVO

Risk factor	Odds ratio for BRVO*	Odds ratio for CRVO*
Factors that increase the risk of RVO		
Hypertension	3.3	2.1
Glaucoma history	2.5	5.4
BMI (age 20) ≥24.4 kg/m²	1.9	
α₂-globulin ≥8.20 g/l	1.7	
CVD	1.6	
Diabetes		1.8
ESR ≥32 (women)		4.4
Antithrombin III > 117		1.8
Factors that decrease the risk of RVO		
Ethanol consumption ≥1 oz daily	0.5	0.6
HDL cholesterol ≥1.81 mmol/l	0.5	
Current estrogen use (women)		0.3
Physically active	0.5	0.5

*adjusted in multiple logistic regression models for age, gender, race, clinic, and all the other variables considered.

Criticisms and Limitations: The majority of individuals in this study (73%–81%) were white; the findings may not be generalizable to other racial/ethnic groups.

The associations of BRVO and CRVO with hypertension and glaucoma might have led to a more rigorous evaluation for these conditions in the cases than the controls, and therefore a bias in the ascertainment of hypertension or glaucoma status. However, when the data were reanalyzed including only patients whose diagnosis of hypertension or glaucoma clearly preceded the time of diagnosis of BRVO/CRVO, hypertension and glaucoma remained significantly associated with risk of BRVO and CRVO.

Some of the nonischemic cases may have been misclassified because they might have eventually converted to the ischemic form; this would have lessened the ability to detect differences in risk factors for the two types of CRVO.

Other Relevant Studies and Information:

- The Eye Disease Case-Control Study also identified 79 cases of hemiretinal vein occlusion (HRVO). Systemic hypertension, history of diabetes mellitus, and history of glaucoma were associated with increased risk of HRVO.[3]

- A case-control study with prospective follow-up to evaluate comorbidity before and after the diagnosis of BRVO found that diabetes, hypertension, and peripheral artery disease are associated with an increased risk of developing branch retinal vein occlusion up to a decade later. Branch retinal vein occlusion was associated with an increased risk of subsequently developing hypertension, diabetes, congestive heart failure, and cerebrovascular disease.[4]
  - Risk factors present 10 years and 1 year before the diagnosis of branch retinal vein occlusion included peripheral artery disease (odds ratio 1.83), diabetes (odds ratio 1.74) and arterial hypertension (odds ratio 2.16).
  - After the diagnosis, patients had an increased risk of developing arterial hypertension (incidence rate ratio 1.37), diabetes (incidence rate ratio 1.51), congestive heart failure (incidence rate ratio 1.41), and cerebrovascular disease (incidence rate ratio 1.49).
- In a meta-analysis, other CRVO associations were various causes of vasculitis, hematologic malignancies, and hypercoagulation.[5]
  - Additionally, it has been suggested that severity of hypertension and/ or diabetes may influence the risk of development of a retinal vein occlusion.
  - African Americans have a 58% increased risk of CRVO compared to whites, and women were 25% less likely than men to have a CRVO.

Summary and Implications: The association of retinal vein occlusion with hypertension, hyperlipidemia, and diabetes should prompt a medical assessment of these and other risk factors for cardiovascular disease. Additionally, patients with BRVO and CRVO should be evaluated for open-angle glaucoma. Diagnosis and treatment of systemic hypertension, weight reduction, increased physical activity, and optimization of serum HDL cholesterol are highly encouraged to reduce risk of developing BRVO and CRVO. In women, postmenopausal estrogen use should be considered.

CLINICAL CASE: AN ELDERLY MAN WITH BRVO

Case History
A 70-year-old Caucasian man with a history of type 2 diabetes, hypertension, obesity, and mild alcohol intake presents to the clinic with sudden onset blurring of vision in the right eye 1 day prior. On exam he is found to have retinal hemorrhages along the superotemporal arcade suggestive of a BRVO. The

patient wants to know what could have caused this condition? Based on the findings of the Eye Disease Case-Control Study, what would you say?

A. Your hypertension and diabetes likely contributed to your condition. It is important to optimize control of your hypertension and diabetes.
B. Your hypertension likely contributed to your condition. It is important to optimize control of your hypertension.
C. Your diabetes likely contributed to your condition. You should have your A1C level checked and discontinue alcohol use immediately.
D. Your consumption of alcohol likely contributed to your condition. You should discontinue alcohol use immediately.

Suggested Answer
Option B.

References

1. Risk factors for branch retinal vein occlusion. The Eye Disease Case-Control Study Group. *Am J Ophthalmol.* 1993;116(3):286–96.
2. Risk factors for central retinal vein occlusion. The Eye Disease Case-Control Study Group. *Arch Ophthalmol.* 1996;114(5):545–54.
3. Sperduto RD, Hiller R, Chew E, et al. Risk factors for hemiretinal vein occlusion: comparison with risk factors for central and branch retinal vein occlusion: the eye disease case-control study. *Ophthalmology.* 1998;105(5):765–71.
4. Bertelsen M, Linneberg A, Rosenberg T, et al. Comorbidity in patients with branch retinal vein occlusion: case-control study. *BMJ.* 2012;345:e7885.
5. Kolar P. Risk factors for central and branch retinal vein occlusion: a meta-analysis of published clinical data. *J Ophthalmol.* 2014;2014:724780.
6. Li J, Paulus YM, Shuai Y, Fang W, Liu Q, Yuan S. New developments in the classification, pathogenesis, risk factors, natural history, and treatment of branch retinal vein occlusion. *J Ophthalmol.* 2017;2017:4936924.

21

Argon Laser Photocoagulation for Macular Edema in Branch Vein Occlusion*

The Branch Vein Occlusion Study (BVOS)

> The Branch Vein Occlusion Study demonstrates that argon laser photocoagulation improves the visual outcome to a significant degree in eyes with branch vein occlusion and visual acuity reduced from macula edema to 20/40 or worse.
>
> —BVOS GROUP[1]

Research Question: Can argon laser photocoagulation improve visual acuity in eyes with branch retinal vein occlusion (BRVO) and macular edema reducing visual acuity to 20/40 or worse?[1]

Funding: National Eye Institute, National Institutes of Health.

Year Study Began: 1977.

Year Study Published: 1984.

Study Location: 5 centers in the United States.

* Basic and Clinical Science Course, Section 12. *Retina and Vitreous*. San Francisco: American Academy of Ophthalmology; 2018–2019: 128–129.

Who Was Studied: Patients with a BRVO occurring 3 to 18 months earlier with best corrected visual acuity (BCVA) of 20/40 or worse from macular edema, confirmation of fovea-involving macular edema on fluorescein angiography, no significant intraretinal hemorrhage limiting safe laser photocoagulation or evaluation by fluorescein angiography, no hemorrhage involving the fovea, and absence of other ocular disease that could limit visual acuity. If it was unclear when onset of BRVO occurred, the presence of segmental intraretinal hemorrhage was considered as evidence of recent occlusion. (Patients with BRVOs less than 3 months in onset were not eligible because some spontaneous improvement in visual acuity was often observed clinically during this period.) If a patient was on anticoagulation for the BRVO, it was discontinued prior to enrollment in the study.

Who Was Excluded: Patients on anticoagulation for systemic conditions who were unable to discontinue medication.

How Many Patients: 139.

Study Overview: The BVOS was a randomized, incompletely masked, controlled clinical trial (Figure 21.1).[1]

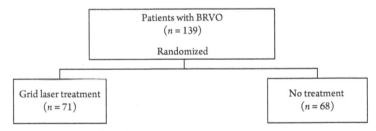

Figure 21.1. Summary of BVOS.

Study Intervention: Patients were recruited into 4 groups of BRVO; certain patients were eligible for placement in more than 1 group. Patients in group 3 (eyes at risk of macular edema, reported in this paper) were randomly allocated either to receive grid laser treatment with the argon laser within the involved macular area or to receive no treatment (control group). (Note: by design, some patients in both the treatment and control groups received scatter laser photocoagulation in other areas of the retina because of the risk of development of neovascularization or vitreous hemorrhage development.)

Follow-Up: Mean follow-up was 3.1 years.

Endpoints: The primary outcome was BCVA.

RESULTS

- Sixty-five percent of eyes treated with laser gained $\geq$ 2 lines from baseline visual acuity (maintained for at least 2 consecutive follow-up visits), compared to 37% of control eyes ($P = .014$).
  - On average, treated eyes gained 1.33 lines of vision compared to 0.23 lines in control eyes ($P < .001$).
  - At 3 years, 60% of eyes in the treatment arm had visual acuities of $\geq$ 20/40, compared to 34% of eyes in the control arm ($P = .02$).
- Although more control group patients were observed to have lost $\geq$ 2 lines of visual acuity (17% vs. 12%), the difference was not statistically significant between groups.
- The probability of increased visual acuity was higher for those not on antihypertensive medication ($P = .09$).
  - The eyes of control patients taking antihypertensive medications fared worse than the nonhypertensive patients (15% vs. 50% respectively for gaining $\geq$ 2 lines on two consecutive visits).
  - However, with laser treatment, 61% of eyes in patients taking antihypertensive medications eyes gained $\geq$ 2 lines of visual acuity (vs. 15% of hypertensive controls) whereas 68% of eyes in patients not taking antihypertensive medications gained vision (vs. 50% of nonhypertensive controls), suggesting that laser treatment is more beneficial for hypertensives than nonhypertensives.
- The probability of increased visual acuity decreased with duration of occlusion ($P = .004$).
  - 70% of eyes were more likely to improve in the first year after initial BRVO compared to 32% of eyes entered after 1 year ($P = .0025$). There was no statistically significant difference between treated and control groups ($P = .92$).

Criticisms and Limitations: The study did not investigate patients with visual acuity >20/40. Thus, the BVOS could not make any recommendations regarding laser treatment in eyes with macular edema and visual acuity better than 20/40.

The study was not designed to evaluate how long after an initial BRVO a patient should be treated. There was no evidence from the BVOS results on whether the timing of laser treatment varies with occlusion duration. (Twenty-two patients [16%] had a duration of BRVO longer than 18 months.)

Eyes with visual loss from intraretinal hemorrhage in the fovea or eyes with nonperfusion of the foveal capillaries were not evaluated. Therefore, no recommendation regarding grid photocoagulation can be made about these patients.

By design, some patients in group III (eyes at risk for macular edema) were also in groups I or II (eyes at risk for neovascularization development or at risk for vitreous hemorrhage development, respectively). Thus, some eyes received scatter photocoagulation in addition to grid photocoagulation. It was assumed that the scatter treatment would not affect the macular edema.

The definition of hypertension used in this study is not the definition used today. This study did not define hypertension by blood pressure measurements, but rather on whether or not a patient was on antihypertensive medications.

Other Relevant Studies and Information:

- A randomized clinical trial comparing 1-mg and 4-mg doses of intravitreal triamcinolone with grid laser photocoagulation in eyes with vision loss associated with macular edema secondary to BRVO found no difference between groups in visual acuity at 12 months; however, rates of adverse events (particularly elevated intraocular pressure and cataract) were highest in the 4-mg group.[2]
- Analysis of pooled data from two identical randomized, sham-controlled clinical trials of dexamethasone intravitreal implant (DEX) in eyes with vision loss due to macular edema associated with BRVO or central retinal vein occlusion (CRVO) showed that at all times patients in the DEX group had a lower percentage of eyes having ≥ 15 lines of visual acuity loss compared to sham group. (This study was limited by the absence of grid laser treatment for the control group.)[3]
- A randomized, sham injection-controlled, double-masked, clinical trial comparing intraocular injections of 0.3 mg or 0.5 mg ranibizumab in patients with macular edema following BRVO found that intraocular injections of 0.3 mg or 0.5 mg ranibizumab provided rapid, effective treatment for macular edema following BRVO with low rates of ocular and nonocular safety events.[4] (See chapter 22.)
- A double-masked, randomized, clinical trial comparing 2-mg intravitreal aflibercept injection (IAI) compared with grid laser in eyes with macular edema after BRVO found that 6 IAI injections every 8 weeks maintained control of macular edema and visual benefits through week 52. In the laser group, rescue IAI given from week 24 onward resulted in substantial visual improvements at week 52.[5]

Summary and Implications: After this study, grid photocoagulation of the macula became the standard of care for BRVO with macular edema with foveal involvement and capillary leakage with visual acuity of 20/40 or worse. Newer treatments such as intravitreal corticosteroids and anti-vascular endothelial growth factor (VEGF) agents (see chapter 22) are under investigation and are increasingly being used "off-label." However, grid laser photocoagulation remains the gold standard therapy for perfused macular edema in BRVO; advantages are that it is proven, widely available, nonsurgical, and of relatively moderate cost. Treatment guidelines currently recommend observation for 3 to 6 months to allow for improved angiographic evaluation of macular edema and capillary nonperfusion; grid laser is recommended for individuals with nonimproving visual acuity of 20/40 or worse due to perfused macular edema.[6]

CLINICAL CASE: A MIDDLE-AGED MAN WITH BRVO

Case History

A 61-year-old man presents to the clinic with complaints of decreased peripheral vision in his left eye. His BCVA is 20/30 in that eye. He is found to have a segmental area of intraretinal hemorrhages along the superotemporal arcade. Fluorescein angiography is consistent with a BRVO. Three months later, he is observed to have a BCVA of 20/50. Fluorescein angiography reveals a new area of macular edema involving the fovea with capillary leakage; optical coherence tomography confirms this. Based on the results of the BVOS, what would be the recommended intervention for this patient?

A. Grid argon laser photocoagulation.
B. Pars plana vitrectomy with endolaser.
C. Observation only.
D. Scatter argon laser photocoagulation.

Suggested Answer

The history and examination findings are suggestive of BRVO. At 3 months, the patient has now developed macular edema with worsening visual acuity. Fluorescein angiography and optical coherence tomography show evidence of cystoid macular edema involving the fovea. Although dexamethasone and ranibizumab are excellent options in treating the cystoid macular edema in this patient, the question asks for the recommended treatment based on the BVOS. Grid photocoagulation of the macula versus observation was evaluated in this study, and there was an improvement of ≥ 2 lines of visual acuity in treated eyes compared to control eyes. Thus, grid photocoagulation is the best option for this patient (option A). In modern clinical practice, intravitreal injection of an anti-VEGF agent or dexamethasone as an initial treatment would be better options than grid photocoagulation for this patien,t based on the results of the GENEVA, CRUISE, and VIBRANT studies.

References

1. Argon laser photocoagulation for macular edema in branch vein occlusion. The Branch Vein Occlusion Study Group. *Am J Ophthalmol.* 1984;98(3):271–82.
2. Scott IU, Ip MS, VanVeldhuisen PC, et al.; SCORE Study Research Group. A randomized trial comparing the efficacy and safety of intravitreal triamcinolone with standard care to treat vision loss associated with macular edema secondary to branch retinal vein occlusion: the Standard Care vs Corticosteroid for Retinal Vein Occlusion (SCORE) study report 6. *Arch Ophthalmol.* 2009;127(9):1115–28.
3. Haller JA, Bandello F, Belfort R Jr, et al.; OZURDEX GENEVA Study Group. Randomized, sham-controlled trial of dexamethasone intravitreal implant in patients with macular edema due to retinal vein occlusion. *Ophthalmology.* 2010;117(6):1134–46.e3.
4. Campochiaro PA, Heier JS, Feiner L, et al.; BRAVO Investigators. Ranibizumab for macular edema following branch retinal vein occlusion: six-month primary end point results of a phase III study. *Ophthalmology.* 2010;117(6):1102–12.e1.
5. Clark WL, Boyer DS, Heier JS, et al. Intravitreal aflibercept for macular edema following branch retinal vein occlusion: 52-week results of the VIBRANT study. *Ophthalmology.* 2016;123(2):330–6.
6. American Academy of Ophthalmology ONE® Network. Branch retinal vein occlusion. Available at https://www.aao.org/focalpointssnippetdetail.aspx?id=4500f02a-755d-446d-97a6-d80fc65833ab. Accessed 4/5/2019.

22

Intraocular Injections of Ranibizumab in Patients with Macular Edema Following Branch Retinal Vein Occlusion[*]

Ranibizumab for Macular Edema Following Branch Retinal Vein Occlusion (BRAVO) Study

Intraocular injections of 0.3 mg or 0.5 mg ranibizumab provided rapid, effective treatment for macular edema following BRVO with low rates of ocular and nonocular safety events.

—BRAVO Study Group[1]

Research Question: What is the safety and efficacy of intraocular injections of 0.3 mg and 0.5 mg ranibizumab in patients with macular edema following branch retinal vein occlusion (BRVO)?[1]

Funding: Genentech (San Francisco, CA).

Year Study Began: 2007.

Year Study Published: 2010.

Study Location: 93 centers in the United States.

---

[*] Basic and Clinical Science Course, Section 12. *Retina and Vitreous*. San Francisco: American Academy of Ophthalmology; 2018–2019: 136.

Who Was Studied: Patients, 18 years of age and older, with macular edema involving the foveal center secondary to BRVO diagnosed within 12 months before study, a best corrected visual acuity (BCVA) 20/40 to 20/400, and mean central subfield thickness ≥250 μm measured on optical coherence tomography (OCT).

Who Was Excluded: Patients with a prior episode of BRVO, a brisk afferent pupillary defect, or >10-letter improvement in BCVA during the 28-day screening period, were ineligible. Other exclusion criteria (listed in Table 1 of the paper) included a history of "dry" or "wet" age-related macular degeneration (AMD), previous panretinal scatter photocoagulation or sector laser photocoagulation within the previous 3 months (or anticipated within 4 months), presence of diabetic retinopathy, or any prior anti–vascular endothelial growth factor (VEGF) treatment in the study or fellow eye within the previous 3 months or systemic anti-VEGF or pro-VEGF within the previous 6 months.

How Many Patients: 397 (1 eye per patient).

Study Overview: The BRAVO study was a 6-month, phase III, randomized, injection-controlled study, with an additional 6 months of follow-up (total 12 months) (Figure 22.1).

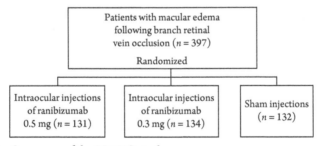

Figure 22.1. Summary of the BRAVO study.

Study Intervention: Patients were randomly allocated to treatment with monthly intraocular injections of either ranibizumab 0.5 mg, ranibizumab 0.3 mg, or sham injection, for 6 months.

Patients were eligible to receive additional monthly injections if needed during the 6-month observation period if BCVA in the study eye was ≤ 20/40 or mean central subfield thickness on optical coherence tomography was ≥ 250 mm. Starting at month 3, patients were eligible for rescue macular grid laser treatment once if hemorrhages had cleared sufficiently and if certain criteria were met: visual acuity ≤20/40 or mean central subfield thickness ≥250 μm, and if the patient had not significantly improved regarding visual acuity or central subfield thickness when compared to 3 months prior.

Follow-Up: 12 months–6 months as an injection-controlled study, with 6 additional months of follow-up.

Endpoint: The primary outcome measure was mean change from baseline best corrected visual acuity (BCVA) at month 6.

RESULTS

- Mean change from baseline BCVA letter score at month 6 was 16.6 and 18.3 in the 0.3 mg and 0.5 mg ranibizumab groups, respectively, and 7.3 in the sham group ($P < .0001$ for each ranibizumab group versus sham).
  - The percentage of patients who gained ≥ 15 letters at month 6 was 55.2% (0.3 mg) and 61.1% (0.5 mg) in the ranibizumab groups and 28.8% and the sham group ($P < .0001$).
  - At month 6, significantly more ranibizumab treated patients (0.3 mg, 67.9%; 0.5 mg 64.9%) had BCVA of ≥20/40 compared with sham patients (41.7%; $P < .0001$).
- Central foveal thickness decreased by a mean of 337 μm (0.3 mg) and 345 μm (0.5 mg) in the ranibizumab groups and 158 μm in the sham group ($P < .0001$).
  - The median percent reduction in excess foveal thickness at month 6 was 97% and 97.6% and the 0.3 mg and 0.5 mg groups, respectively, and 27.9% in the sham group.
- More patients in the sham group (54.5%) received rescue grid laser compared with the 0.3 mg (18.7%) and 0.5 mg (19.8%) ranibizumab groups.
- The safety profile was consistent with previous ranibizumab trials.

Criticism and Limitations: The short duration of the study (12 months total) precluded investigating what percentage of patients remained edema-free after ranibizumab treatment was discontinued, or whether treatment with ranibizumab after a 6-month delay would allow the sham group to achieve similar visual outcomes to those seen in the ranibizumab groups at 12 months. If macular edema recurs, can ranibizumab-induced visual gains be maintained with further treatment?

The BRAVO study did not directly compare the efficacy of ranibizumab injections and grid laser treatment for macular edema following BRVO, in part because they are very different types of treatment.

More than 80% of study participants were white; the generalizability of the results to other racial/ethnic groups is uncertain.

Other Relevant Studies and Information:

• Analysis of pooled data from two identical randomized, sham-controlled clinical trials of dexamethasone intravitreal implant (DEX) in eyes with vision loss due to macular edema associated with BRVO or central retinal vein occlusion (CRVO) showed that at all times patients in the DEX group had a lower percentage of eyes having ≥ 15 lines of visual acuity loss compared to sham group.[2] (This study was limited by the absence of grid laser treatment for the control group.)

• The HORIZON Trial was an open-label year-long extension of BRAVO. In this study, patients were seen at least every 3 months and given 0.5 mg ranibizumab if mean central foveal thickness was ≥250 μm or if there was persistent macular edema affecting the patient's visual acuity. Investigators found that the injection burden decreased compared to year 1 and visual acuity gains were maintained.[3]

• The VIBRANT study was first trial to compare anti-VEGF therapy (aflibercept was used in the study) directly with laser and the results were strongly in favor of aflibercept with similar side-effect profiles in both groups.[4]

• A double-masked, randomized, clinical trial comparing 2 mg intravitreal aflibercept injection (IAI) compared with grid laser in eyes with macular edema after BRVO found that 6 IAI injections every 8 weeks maintained control of macular edema and visual benefits through week 52. In the laser group, rescue IAI given from week 24 onward resulted in substantial visual improvements at week 52.[5]

Summary and Implications: The study clearly demonstrated that 6 monthly injections of ranibizumab provided visual benefit to patients with macular edema following BRVO. This study helped direct the paradigm shift towards anti-VEGF agents as the first-line treatment for macular edema secondary to BRVO.

CLINICAL CASE: AN ELDERLY MAN WITH MACULAR EDEMA FOLLOWING BRVO

Case History

A 73-year-old white man presents to your clinic complaining of blurring of vision in the right eye which started suddenly 2 weeks ago and has continued to worsen slightly. On examination his visual acuity is 20/100 in the right eye and 20/25 and the left eye. Confrontation visual fields are full in both eyes and there is no relative afferent pupillary defect. His retinal exam is unremarkable aside from tortuosity and engorgement of the vein draining the superotemporal quadrant, with dot-blot hemorrhages and two cotton wool spots along the superotemporal arcade. There is also central macular edema with retinal hemorrhages. There is no retinal neovascularization or vitreous hemorrhage. Fluorescein angiography (FA) and optical coherence tomography confirm the presence of a nonischemic BRVO in the right eye with macula edema. Based on the results of the BRAVO clinical trial, what do you recommend to the patient as the best initial treatment option for visual recovery?

A. Intraocular injection of DEX.
B. Intraocular injection of anti-VEGF (e.g., ranibizumab).
C. Macular grid laser.
D. Topical prednisolone acetate 1% drops 4 times daily.

Suggested Answer

The history and examination findings in this patient are typical for the development of macular edema secondary to a branch retinal vein occlusion. Based on the results of the BRAVO study, this patient should be treated with an anti-VEGF agent (option B) given intraocularly after a thorough discussion of the risks, benefits, and alternatives. The patient needs to understand that future intraocular injections will also be needed if he is to follow the initial BRAVO protocol. Also, there is the possibility of needing a future laser procedure in the event the macular edema does not respond or if the patient develops neovascularization.

References

1. Campochiaro PA, Heier JS, Feiner L, et al.; BRAVO Investigators. Ranibizumab for macular edema following branch retinal vein occlusion: six-month primary end point results of a phase III study. *Ophthalmology*. 2010;117(6):1102–12.e1.

2. Haller JA, Bandello F, Belfort R Jr, et al.; OZURDEX GENEVA Study Group. Randomized, sham-controlled trial of dexamethasone intravitreal implant in patients with macular edema due to retinal vein occlusion. *Ophthalmology*. 2010;117(6):1134–1146.e3.

3. Heier JS, Campochiaro PA, Yau L, et al. Ranibizumab for macular edema due to retinal vein occlusion: long-term follow-up in the HORIZON Trial. *Ophthalmology*. 2012;119(4):802–9.

4. Campochiaro PA, Clark WL, Boyer DS, et al. Intravitreal aflibercept for macular edema following branch retinal vein occlusion: the 24-week results of the VIBRANT study. *Ophthalmology*. 2015;122(3):538–44.

5. Clark WL, Boyer DS, Heier JS, et al. Intravitreal aflibercept for macular edema following branch retinal vein occlusion: 52-week results of the VIBRANT Study. *Ophthalmology*. 2016;123(2):330–6.

23

Grid Pattern Photocoagulation for Macular Edema in Central Vein Occlusion[*]

The Central Vein Occlusion Study (CVOS)

> Overall, visual acuity results in the CVOS were not different for treated and control eyes. Therefore, we do not recommend grid pattern argon laser photocoagulation for macula edema due to central vein occlusion, based on the CVOS eligibility and treatment protocols.
>
> —CENTRAL VEIN OCCLUSION STUDY GROUP[1]

Research Question: Does treatment with macular grid photocoagulation improve or preserve visual acuity in eyes with macular edema involving the fovea secondary to central retinal vein occlusion (CRVO) with best corrected visual acuity of 20/50 or worse?[1]

Funding: National Eye Institute, National Institutes of Health.

Year Study Began: 1988.

Year Study Published: 1995.

Study Location: 8 clinics in the United States and 1 in France.

---

[*] Basic and Clinical Science Course, Section 12. *Retina and Vitreous*. San Francisco: American Academy of Ophthalmology; 2018–2019: 130–135.

Who Was Studied: Patients with nonischemic CRVO of at least 3 months duration, central macular edema with foveal involvement based on fluorescein angiography, visual acuity ranging from 5/200 to 20/50 (with no other pathological causes explaining decreased vision), and no spontaneous improvement in visual acuity on two repeated visits spaced 2 weeks apart prior to enrollment.

Who Was Excluded: Patients were excluded if nonperfusion was present in the macula. Patients were ineligible if they had prior laser treatment for other retinal vascular disease in the affected eye, coexisting eye disease with potential to affect visual acuity over the course of the study, presence of any retinal vascular disease including diabetic retinopathy in either eye, branch arterial or vein occlusion (new or old) in affected eye, neovascularization of the retina in the affected eye, or presence of a vitreous hemorrhage (breakthrough hemorrhage was allowed).

How Many Patients: 155 (1 eye per patient).

Study Overview: The Central Vein Occlusion Study was a randomized, controlled, clinical trial (Figure 22.1).[1-4]

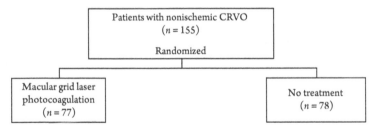

Figure 23.1. Summary of CVOS.

Study Intervention: Patients were randomly allocated to macular grid photocoagulation with the argon green laser or to observation only. If improvement in visual acuity at 4 months or at the annual follow-up was 9 letters or less and treatable macular edema was present angiographically, the patient was scheduled for retreatment; 23 of the 77 required retreatment after 4 months; and of these, 4 more required additional treatment.

Follow-Up: Maximum 3 years (88/155 completed 3 years of follow-up).

Endpoints: The primary outcome measure was visual acuity.

RESULTS

- Initial median visual acuity was 20/160 in treated eyes and 20/125 in control eyes; final median visual acuity was 20/200 in treated eyes and 20/160 in control eyes. The mean changes in visual acuity score from baseline to the 36-month visit was a loss of 4 letters in treated eyes and a 3-letter loss in untreated eyes.
- There was no statistically significant difference between treated and untreated eyes in visual acuity at any point during follow-up.
  - Thirty-three percent (25/75) of treated eyes and 29% (22/77) of untreated eyes lost at least 2 lines of vision (10 letters) between baseline and the final follow-up visit.
  - Twenty-three percent (17/75) of treated eyes and 18% (14/77) of untreated eyes improved by 2 or more lines.
- There was no statistically significant difference between treated and untreated groups in change in visual acuity when stratified by duration of CRVO (duration less than 1 year, or 1 year or more).
- In the treatment group, visual acuity tended to worsen in patients aged >60 and to improve in younger patients, but this difference was not statistically significant ($P = .49$).
  - In the treatment group, 17 patients had improvement in visual acuity; 11/17 of these eyes came from the subgroup of treated and untreated patients younger than 60 years of age.
- Treatment with macular grid photocoagulation greatly decreased the amount of macular edema observed on fluorescein angiography. At 12 months, no macular edema was observed in 31% of treated eyes, whereas all untreated eyes had some degree of macula edema ($P < .0001$).
  - In patients with CRVO < 1 year duration, 42% of treated eyes had measurable macula edema at 24 months compared to 94% of untreated eyes ($P < .0001$). In patients with CRVO of 1 year or longer, 42% of treated eyes had measurable macular edema at 24 months compared with 95% of untreated eyes ($P < .0001$).
  - The qualitative improvement in macular edema was assessed by comparing intensity of leakage on fluorescein angiography at first follow-up visit at 4 months compared to the initial angiogram. Forty-eight percent of treated eyes demonstrated improvement, 41% were stable, and 12% worsened; 18% of untreated eyes demonstrated improvement, 66% were stable, and 16% worsened ($P < .001$).

Criticisms and Limitations: In the CVOS macular edema was judged using the fluorescein angiogram; optical coherence tomography (OCT), now regarded as the gold standard for assessment and management of patients with RVO, was not available.

There was a suggestion that patients younger than 60 years of age benefited from treatment, but unfortunately the study did not have enough power to determine statistical significance.

More than 90% of patients were white, which may limit the generalizability of the findings.

Other Relevant Studies and Information:

- In recent years there has been a paradigm shift in the management of macular edema secondary to CRVO; new treatment options include intravitreal anti–vascular endothelial growth factor (VEGF) agents and corticosteroids. See chapter 24.

Summary and Implications: This study showed that macular grid photocoagulation had no place in the treatment of macular edema in nonischemic CRVOs; at that time the standard of care continued to be observation. Treatment with intravitreal anti-VEGF agents is now the standard of care.

CLINICAL CASE: A MIDDLE AGED MAN WITH CRVO

Case History

A 61-year-old man with hypertension and diabetes mellitus presents to the clinic with complaints of sudden loss of vision in his right eye. His visual acuity is 20/50 in that eye. He is found to have 4 quadrants of retinal hemorrhage with dilated and engorged vessels in his right eye. Three months later his visual acuity in the right eye has decreased to 20/100. Fluorescein angiography reveals nonischemic CRVO with macula edema. OCT of the macula confirms cystoid macular edema. Based on the results of the CVOS Group M report, what would be the recommended intervention for this patient?

A. Intravitreal dexamethasone implant.
B. Macular grid photocoagulation.
C. Observation.
D. Panretinal photocoagulation.

Suggested Answer

The patient has a nonischemic CRVO with cystoid macular edema. Although dexamethasone and ranibizumab are excellent options in treating the cystoid macular edema in this patient, the question asks for the recommended treatment based on the CVOS study. Macular grid photocoagulation versus observation was evaluated in this study, and there was no statistically significant difference between the treated and untreated group. Thus, observation (option C) would be the best choice for this question. In modern clinical practice, both dexamethasone and ranibizumab would be better options than observation for this patient based on the results of the GENEVA and CRUISE studies.

References

1. Evaluation of grid pattern photocoagulation for macular edema in central vein occlusion. The Central Vein Occlusion Study Group M report. *Ophthalmology.* 1995;102(10):1425–33.
2. Baseline and early natural history report. The Central Vein Occlusion Study. *Arch Ophthalmol.* 1993;111(8):1087–95.
3. Central vein occlusion study of photocoagulation therapy: baseline findings. Central Vein Occlusion Study Group. *Online J Curr Clin Trials.* 1993;Doc No 95.
4. Central vein occlusion study of photocoagulation: manual of operations. Central Vein Occlusion Study Group. *Online J Curr Clin Trials.* 1993;Doc No 92.

24

Steroids in the Treatment of Central Retinal Vein Occlusion*

The Standard Care vs. Corticosteroid for Retinal Vein Occlusion (SCORE-CRVO) Study

Based on the results of the SCORE-CRVO trial, intravitreal triamcinolone in a 1-mg dose and following the retreatment criteria used in this study should be considered for up to 1 year, and possibly 2 years, in patients with vision loss associated with macular edema secondary to CRVO who have characteristics similar to the participants studied in this trial.

—SCORE STUDY RESEARCH GROUP[1]

Research Question: What is the efficacy and safety of intravitreal triamcinolone (IVT) compared to observation in eyes with vision loss associated with macular edema due to perfused (nonischemic) central retinal vein occlusion (CRVO)?[1]

Funding: National Eye Institute, National Institutes of Health.

Year Study Began: 2004.

Year Study Published: 2009.

* Basic and Clinical Science Course, Section 12. *Retina and Vitreous.* San Francisco: American Academy of Ophthalmology; 2018–2019: 137–138.

Study Location: 84 clinics in the United States.

Who Was Studied: Patients with center-involved macular edema due to per-fused (nonischemic) CRVO and mean central subfield retinal thickness ≥250 μm, with a best corrected visual acuity between 20/40 and 20/400.

Who Was Excluded: Patients were excluded from the study if they had mac-ular edema due to other causes or other ocular conditions that could limit visual acuity improvement, including a visually significant cataract. Patients with prior treatment with intravitreal corticosteroids or peribulbar steroid injection within 6 months prior to randomization were also ineligible, as were those with a history of focal or grid macular photocoagulation within 15 weeks or panretinal photo-coagulation within 4 months prior to randomization.

How Many Patients: 271 (1 eye per participant).

Study Overview: The SCORE Study was a prospective, randomized clinical trial (Figure 24.1).[1]

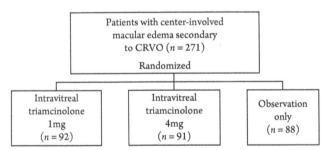

Figure 24.1. Summary of the SCORE-CRVO study.

Study Intervention: Patients were randomly assigned to receive standard care (observation group), 1 mg of IVT, or 4 mg of IVT, with retreatment at 4-month intervals if needed. Eyes assigned to observation could receive IVT when there was a loss from baseline in best corrected visual acuity letter score of 15 or more at 2 consecutive 4-month-interval visits, as a result of persistent or recurrent macular edema.

Follow-up: 1 year.

Endpoints: The proportion of participants who experienced a gain in visual acuity letter score of 15 or more from baseline to month 12.

RESULTS

- Prior to month 12, the average number of injections was similar in the triamcinolone groups, with 2.2 in the 1-mg triamcinolone group and 2.0 in the 4-mg triamcinolone group.
- 26.5% in the 1-mg triamcinolone group and 25.6% in the 4-mg triamcinolone group achieved visual improvement of 15 or more letters by month 12, compared to 6.8% in the observation group.
  - The odds ratio (OR) for a gain in visual acuity letter score of 15 or more (after adjusting for baseline visual acuity) comparing the 1-mg and 4-mg triamcinolone groups, respectively, with the observation group, were 5.0 ($P = .001$) and 5.0 ($P = .001$).
  - The OR for a gain in visual acuity letter score of 15 or more (after adjusting for baseline visual acuity) comparing the 1-mg with the 4-mg triamcinolone group was 1.0 ($P = .97$).
- Both triamcinolone groups had a similar change from baseline to month 12 in mean visual acuity letter score (an approximately 1- to 2-letter loss) compared with a mean loss of 12 in the observation group.
  - At all time points through 12 months, mean visual acuity was better in the triamcinolone groups than in the observation group.
  - At month 24, a loss in visual acuity letter score of 15 or more (Figure 2B in the paper) was noted in approximately 48% of participants in the observation group compared with approximately 30% of participants in the triamcinolone groups ($P = .06$).
- Each group showed a decrease (measured by optical coherence tomography) in central retinal thickness from baseline, but there was no significant difference between the groups after 1 year.
  - By the scheduled follow-up visit, the percentage of participants with a central retinal thickness of less than 250 μm was similar for the 3 study groups, with the exception of the month 4 visit, at which a greater percentage of participants in the 4-mg triamcinolone group had such a decrease ($P = .002$).
- The rates of cataract formation or progression by month 12 were higher in the 1-mg and 4-mg groups (26% and 33%, respectively) compared to the observation group (18%).
  - 4 eyes in the 4-mg group received cataract surgery by month 12, compared to no eyes in the observation or 1-mg triamcinolone groups.
  - Cataract surgery was more frequent between months 12 and 24 in the 4-mg group, with 21 eyes receiving cataract surgery compared with 3 in the 1-mg group and 0 in the observation group.

- More eyes in the treatment groups (20% in 1-mg group, 35% in the 4-mg group) required IOP-lowering medication over 12 months, compared to 8% in observation eyes.

Criticisms and Limitations: Complete long-term follow-up data were lacking, as only about half of participants were assessed at month 24. This made it difficult to evaluate the effects on IOP and cataract. From the data available between month 12 and 2 years, the beneficial effect of both doses of IVT on visual acuity attenuated between 12 months and 2 years, possibly because of cataract development/progression.

This study was limited to nonischemic CRVOs with macular perfusion, and the findings cannot be extrapolated to ischemic CRVOs. Furthermore, only one steroid was tested, and different classes of steroid may give different results.

More than 80% of patients were white, which may limit the generalizability of the findings.

Other Relevant Studies and Information:

- In recent years there has been a paradigm shift in the management of macular edema secondary to CRVO; new treatment options include intravitreal anti–vascular endothelial growth factor (VEGF) agents and corticosteroids.
  - In several recent systematic reviews/meta-analyses, aflibercept, bevacizumab, and ranibizumab showed greater improvement in visual acuity and reduction in central retinal thickness than sham/placebo treatment. Aflibercept may have a slight advantage over ranibizumab, particularly for the management of persistent macular edema.[2-4] Clinical trials are ongoing.
  - Intravitreal steroids are now used much less frequently; however, they may have a role in resistant cases, alone or in combination with anti-VEGFs.[5,6]

Summary and implications: The SCORE-CRVO Study was the first to establish an effective treatment for perfused CRVO; the results suggested that intravitreal triamcinolone in a 1-mg dose should be considered for up to 1 year, and possibly 2 years, in patients with vision loss associated with macular edema secondary to CRVO. However, even with treatment, by 12 months three-quarters of eyes did not have a gain in visual acuity of 15 or more letters, and one-quarter had a loss of visual acuity of 15 or more letters. Treatment with intravitreal anti-VEGF agents has been shown to produce greater improvement in visual acuity and is now the standard of care.

CLINICAL CASE: A MIDDLE AGED MAN WITH CRVO

Case History
A 62-year-old African American man presents to the clinic with a 1-week history of blurring of vision in the right eye. The medical history is significant for hypertension and hyperlipidemia. He is a 2 pack a day current smoker. His best corrected visual acuity is 20/100 in the right eye and 20/30 in the left. Anterior segment exam and intraocular pressure are normal in both eyes. Dilated fundus examination of the right eye is suggestive of a CRVO. Dilated examination of the left eye is largely unremarkable with the exception of arteriolar attenuation. A fluorescein angiogram confirms a nonischemic CRVO in the right eye. Optical coherence tomography showed cystoid macular edema with significant thickening. Based on the SCORE-CRVO study, what treatment option would be most beneficial for this patient?

A. Intravitreal avastin.
B. Observation only.
C. Intravitreal triamaclinone 1mg.
D. Intravitreal triamaclinone 4 mg.

Suggested Answer
While intravitreal anti-VEGF agents have largely replaced steroids for the initial treatment of macular edema associated with CRVO, these agents were not studied in the SCORE study. Based on the SCORE study, the best treatment option would be C. The 4-mg dosage was shown to have significantly more side effects and would not be the most appropriate starting therapy.

References

1. Ip MS, Scott IU, VanVeldhuisen PC, et al.; SCORE Study Research Group. A randomized trial comparing the efficacy and safety of intravitreal triamcinolone with observation to treat vision loss associated with macular edema secondary to central retinal vein occlusion: the Standard Care vs Corticosteroid for Retinal Vein Occlusion (SCORE) study report 5. *Arch Ophthalmol.* 2009;127(9):1101–14.
2. Sangroongruangsri S, Ratanapakorn T, Wu O, Anothaisintawee T, Chaikledkaew U. Comparative efficacy of bevacizumab, ranibizumab, and aflibercept for treatment of

macular edema secondary to retinal vein occlusion: a systematic review and network meta-analysis. *Expert Rev Clin Pharmacol.* 2018;11(9):903–16.

3. Qian T, Zhao M, Wan Y, Li M, Xu X. Comparison of the efficacy and safety of drug therapies for macular edema secondary to central retinal vein occlusion. *BMJ Open.* 2018;8(12):e022700.

4. Spooner K, Hong T, Bahrami B, Chang A. A meta-analysis of patients with treatment-resistant macular oedema secondary to retinal vein occlusions following switching to aflibercept. *Acta Ophthalmol.* 2019;97(1):15–23.

5. Ashraf M, Souka AA. Steroids in central retinal vein occlusion: is there a role in current treatment practice? *J Ophthalmol.* 2015;2015:594615.

6. Ashraf M, Souka AA, Singh RP. Central retinal vein occlusion: modifying current treatment protocols. *Eye (Lond).* 2016;30(4):505–14.

25

Cryotherapy for Retinopathy of Prematurity*

Cryotherapy for Retinopathy of Prematurity (CRYO-ROP) Study

At a 3-month assessment, cryotherapy is significantly beneficial for eyes with ROP at a defined threshold level of severity.
— CRYO-ROP Cooperative Group[1]

Research Question: Is cryotherapy effective in reducing the unfavorable ocular outcomes from threshold retinopathy of prematurity (ROP)?[1]

Funding: National Eye Institute, National Institutes of Health.

Year Study Began: 1986.

Year Study Published: 1990.

Study Location: 23 centers in the United States.

Who Was Studied: Infants who weighed less than 1251 g at birth and who developed threshold ROP in at least one eye, defined as 5 or more contiguous or 8 cumulative 30-degree sectors (clock hours) of stage 3 ROP in zone 1 or 2 with plus (+) disease (dilatation and tortuosity of the retinal blood vessels in the posterior pole). Threshold ROP carries a risk of approximately 50% for retinal detachment.

* Basic and Clinical Science Course, Section 6. *Pediatric Ophthalmology and Strabismus.* San Francisco: American Academy of Ophthalmology, 2018–2019: 326–32.

Three-quarters of the infants ("early-entry") had been followed up prospectively from age 1 month; the other quarter were "late-entry," referred with suspected threshold ROP.

Who Was Excluded: If ROP in either eye reached stage 4 (retinal detachment), the infant was considered monocular and deemed ineligible for enrollment.

How Many Patients: 291.

Study Overview: The Multicenter Trial of Cryotherapy for Retinopathy of Prematurity (CRYO-ROP) was a randomized, controlled, interventional clinical trial (Figure 25.1).[1,2]

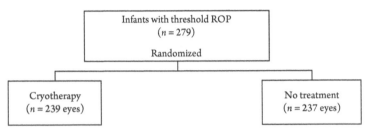

Figure 25.1. Summary of the CRYO-ROP study.

Study Intervention: In the "early entry" infants, initial ophthalmologic examinations began at 4 to 6 weeks of age; "late-entry" infants were examined within 24 hours. If both eyes developed threshold ROP concurrently (bilateral threshold group; $n = 240$), one eye was randomly assigned to receive cryotherapy, while the other eye was allowed to follow its natural course and serve as a control. If the disease in only one eye was confirmed to be at the threshold level (asymmetric group; $n = 51$), only that eye would enter the randomized trial, as an asymmetric case, and it would be randomized to either cryotherapy or no treatment.

Transscleral cryotherapy was applied to the entire circumference of the avascular retina anterior to the ridge. Treatment did not extend posteriorly to the ridge or anteriorly into the pars plana.

Follow-Up: 3 months (preliminary data for 12 months are also presented).

Endpoints: The primary outcome measure was an unfavorable outcome (based on masked grading of photographs taken at the 3-month and 12-month follow-up examinations), defined as (1) a posterior retinal fold, usually involving macula; (2) a retinal detachment involving zone 1 of the posterior pole; or (3) retrolental tissue or "mass" that obscures the view of the posterior pole. All eyes with other fundus appearances were classified as having a favorable outcome. The 12-month exam also measured visual function with preferential-looking techniques.

RESULTS

- The mean gestational age was 26.3 weeks. All patients weighed less than 1251 g at birth; overall, the mean birth weight was 800 g.
  - By the time of randomization and cryotherapy, the infants had gained slightly more than 1000 g from their original birth weight, for a mean weight of 1838 g at the time of cryotherapy.
- The percentage of infants with bilateral threshold disease was 82.5%.
- Whereas 51.4% of control eyes had an unfavorable outcome, this was significantly less frequent in the eyes that received cryotherapy (31.1%) (P < .00001).
- In infants with bilateral threshold retinopathy, 53.0% of control eyes had an unfavorable outcome compared to 31.5% of treated eyes.
  - In infants with asymmetrical disease, 33.3% of control eyes had an unfavorable outcome compared to 27.3% of treated eyes.
- The ocular findings at 3 months in infants with bilateral threshold ROP showed significantly less incidence of synechiae, abnormal pupillary light reaction, shallow anterior chamber, extensive vitreous membranes, total retinal detachment and preretinal membranes in treated eyes compared to control eyes. Conjunctival/episcleral (epibulbar) hyperemia was the only finding in which the treated eyes had a higher event rate than the control eyes ($P = .05$).
- Complications during cryotherapy included conjunctival or subconjunctival hematomas in 11.7% of eyes and unintended conjunctival laceration in 5.3% of eyes. Retinal, preretinal, and vitreous hemorrhage was noted in 22.3% of cases. Transient closure of the central retinal artery was noted in one instance and inadvertent freezing to an area outside of a target zone occurred in two cases. Other events included one case of retinal break and one case of dilation of the tunica vasculosa lentis during treatment.

Criticisms and Limitations: The study design required staging by strict clinical criteria; the nature of the disease and its rapid progression did not allow masked photographic interpretation prior to randomization. A second examination by a different clinician was used as a measure to control for bias in staging.

The interpretation of the results of this study is limited to the benefit of treatment at the defined threshold. It is possible that treatment at an earlier stage may also have been effective in some cases, and this is the subject of a subsequent, second-generation study of laser panretinal photocoagulation for ROP, the Early Treatment for Retinopathy of Prematurity trial (ETROP).

The method of treatment used in the study, peripheral retinal transscleral cryotherapy, was the form of retinal ablation most widely used at that time for treatment for ROP. Subsequently, the wide availability of portable lasers with indirect ophthalmoscopic delivery, which have fewer associated local and systemic adverse effects, including pain and swelling, and do not require conjunctival incision, allowed laser photocoagulation to become the most widely used method of ROP treatment.

Unfavorable anatomic outcomes correlate with severe vision loss, but "favorable" anatomic outcome does not mean normal vision. The choice of anatomic rather than functional outcome may have overestimated the treatment benefit.

Other Relevant Studies and Information:

- At 10 years (247 children examined), eyes that had received cryotherapy were much less likely than control eyes to be blind.[3]
  - Both functional and structural primary outcomes showed fewer unfavorable outcomes in treated vs. control eyes: 44.4% vs. 62.1% ($P < .001$) for distance visual acuity and 27.2% vs. 47.9% ($P < .001$) for fundus status. Near acuity results were similar to those for distance (42.5% vs. 61.6%; $P < .001$). Total retinal detachments had continued to occur in control eyes, increasing from 38.6% at 5 years to 41.4% at 10 years, while treated eyes remained stable (at 22.0%).
- At 15 years (254 surviving children), the benefit of cryotherapy, for both structure and visual function, was maintained.[4]
  - Thirty percent of treated eyes and 51.9% of control eyes ($P < .001$) had unfavorable structural outcomes. Between 10 and 15 years of age, new retinal folds, detachments, or obscuring of the view of the posterior pole occurred in 4.5% of treated and 7.7% of control eyes. Unfavorable visual acuity outcomes were found in 44.7% of treated and 64.3% of control eyes ($P < .001$).

Summary and Implications: The findings of the CRYO-ROP study led to the implementation of neonatal screening and peripheral retinal ablation for acute ROP throughout the United States and beyond. It is difficult to overestimate the impact of this well-designed trial in taking the concept of ablative treatment from controversial to near universal acceptance within a short period of time. In addition to treatment of threshold ROP, the CRYO-ROP study collected the natural history and epidemiologic data that permitted evidence-based screening for ROP. These guidelines have evolved based on subsequent studies, but the basic CRYO-ROP epidemiological data remain the foundation of the existing clinical guidelines for examination of premature infants. Long-term results of CRYO-ROP have also influenced the management of affected patients throughout the remainder of childhood, including long-term surveillance for late retinal changes, refractive error, and amblyopia management.

CLINICAL CASE: A PREMATURE INFANT WITH ROP IN BOTH EYES

Case History

A female infant was born at 26 weeks gestation with a birth weight of 950 g. The Apgar score was 6 at birth and 8 five minutes later. Assisted ventilation was immediately started with 100% oxygen and continued for 3 weeks with an FiO2 (fraction inspiratory oxygen) of 25%. The partial pressure of oxygen (PO2) was maintained at 50–70 mm Hg, but there were three short episodes of PO2 above 100 mm Hg. Examination performed at 2 weeks revealed remnants of tunica vasculosa lentis with normal anterior segments. The fundus examination showed extension of the retinal vessels to zone I. Two weeks later examination of the left eye showed congestion of posterior retinal vessels and severe active ROP (stage III) in zone I–II, 360 degrees. The right eye showed stage 3 ROP in Zone 2 from 1 o'clock to 4 o'clock with no congestion of vessels. What do you recommend to the parents as the best treatment option for her according to the CRYO-ROP trial?

A. Repeat exam in 1 week in both eyes.
B. Cryotherapy of right eye.
C. Cryotherapy of left eye.
D. Cryotherapy of both eyes.

Suggested Answer

The findings in this patient show ROP in both eyes but with the left eye reaching the threshold for treatment according to the CRYO-ROP trial. Based on the findings of this trial, the correct option would be to treat the left eye alone with cryotherapy and monitor the right eye for progression or resolution (option C).

References

1. Cryotherapy for Retinopathy of Prematurity Cooperative Group. Multicenter trial of cryotherapy for retinopathy of prematurity: three-month outcome. *Arch Ophthalmol.* 1990;108(2):195–204.
2. Cryotherapy for Retinopathy of Prematurity Cooperative Group. Multicenter trial of cryotherapy for retinopathy of prematurity: preliminary results. *Arch Ophthalmol.* 1988;106(4):471–9.
3. Cryotherapy for Retinopathy of Prematurity Cooperative Group. Multicenter trial of cryotherapy for retinopathy of prematurity: ophthalmological outcomes at 10 years. *Arch Ophthalmol.* 2001;119(8):1110–8.
4. Palmer EA, Hardy RJ, Dobson V, et al.; Cryotherapy for Retinopathy of Prematurity Cooperative Group. 15-year outcomes following threshold retinopathy of prematurity: final results from the multicenter trial of cryotherapy for retinopathy of prematurity. *Arch Ophthalmol.* 2005;123(3):311–8.

26

Supplemental Therapeutic Oxygen for Prethreshold Retinopathy of Prematurity*

The Supplemental Therapeutic Oxygen for Prethreshold Retinopathy of Prematurity (STOP-ROP) Trial

Use of supplemental oxygen at pulse oximetry saturations of 96% to 99% did not cause additional progression of prethreshold ROP but also did not significantly reduce the number of infants requiring peripheral ablative surgery.

—STOP-ROP MULTICENTER STUDY GROUP[1]

Research Question: In premature infants, does supplemental therapeutic oxygen reduce the probability of progression from prethreshold to threshold ROP and the need for peripheral retinal ablation?

Funding: National Eye Institute, National Institute of Child Health and Human Development, National Institute of Nursing Research, and several National Institutes of Health General Clinical Research Centers, National Institutes of Health; also local funding sources at many centers.

Year Study Began: 1994.

Year Study Published: 2000.

* Basic and Clinical Science Course, Section 12. *Retina and Vitreous.* San Francisco: American Academy of Ophthalmology; 2018–2019.

Study Location: 30 centers in the United States.

Who Was Studied: Premature infants with confirmed prethreshold ROP in at least 1 eye and median pulse oximetry <94% saturation. Prethreshold ROP was defined as: (1) Zone II: any number of clock hours of stage 3 ROP, less than threshold severity, or any stage 2 ROP with at least 2 quadrants of posterior pole dilation/tortuosity disease (plus disease); (2) Zone I: any ROP less than threshold severity.

Who Was Excluded: Patients were excluded if they had pulse oximetry saturation greater than 94% breathing room air, had lethal anomalies, or had congenital anomalies of the eye.

How Many Patients: 649.

Study Overview: The STOP-ROP Trial was a randomized, controlled clinical trial (Figure 26.1).[1]

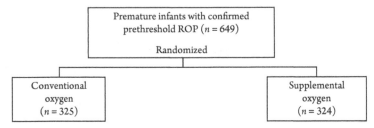

Figure 26.1 Summary of STOP-ROP.

Study Intervention: Infants were randomized to receive supplemental oxygen therapy with pulse oximetry targeted at 96%–99% oxygen saturation or conventional oxygen therapy with pulse oximetry targeted at 89%–94% oxygen saturation for at least 2 weeks.

Follow-Up: Infants were followed to 3 months corrected age (that is, 3 months past the term due date of 40 weeks' postmenstrual age [PMA]).

Endpoints: The primary outcome was the proportion of infants with at least 1 eye progressing to confirmed threshold ROP. An adverse ophthalmic endpoint was defined as reaching threshold criteria for laser or cryotherapy in at least 1 study eye. A favorable ophthalmic endpoint was regression of the ROP into zone 3 for at least 2 consecutive weekly examinations or full retinal vascularization. Ophthalmic outcomes at 3 months' corrected age were classified as: (1)

unfavorable when there were findings of total or partial retinal detachment or when the visual axis was otherwise obstructed, (2) indeterminate when there was macular ectopia, or (3) favorable when there were only minor peripheral findings, laser or cryotherapy scars, or active ROP in zone II or III.

RESULTS

- Enrollment and randomization occurred at an average PMA of 35.4 weeks (range: 30–48 weeks).
- In the supplemental arm, the average oxygen concentration in the 24 hours after randomization increased from 36% ± 14% pretreatment to 46% ± 20%, 24 hours after randomization for those infants on a ventilator, continuous positive airway pressure (CPAP), or hood oxygen; for infants on nasal cannula, the average increase was estimated to be 9.5% ± 16.5%. In the conventional arm, the average oxygen concentration increased from 36% ± 17% to 32% ± 15% in the infants on a ventilator, CPAP, or hood oxygen, and from 28% ± 10% to 26% ± 11% in the nasal cannula infants.
  - During the first 2 weeks, only 8.0% of median saturations for infants assigned to the conventional arm were in the supplemental range or higher, and only 1.8% of median saturations of infants assigned to supplemental therapy were in the conventional range or lower.
- The rate of progression to threshold in at least 1 eye was 48% in the conventional arm and 41% in the supplemental arm ($P = .06$).
  - The same pattern was observed according to severity or zone of baseline ROP.
    - In infants with high severity ROP, the rate of progression to threshold in at least 1 eye was 55% in the conventional arm and 46% in the supplemental arm (not statistically significant). In infants with low-severity ROP, the rate of progression to threshold in at least 1 eye was 46% in the conventional arm and 39% in the supplemental arm (not statistically significant).
    - In infants with zone I ROP, the rate of progression to threshold in at least 1 eye was 56% in the conventional arm and 49% in the supplemental arm (not statistically significant). In infants with zone II ROP, the rate of progression to threshold in at least 1 eye was 46% in the conventional arm and 37% in the supplemental arm (not statistically significant).
    - In infants without plus disease, the rate of progression to threshold in at least 1 eye was 46% in the conventional arm and 32% in the supplemental arm ($P = .004$). In infants with plus disease, the rate of

progression to threshold in at least 1 eye was 52% in the conventional arm and 57% in the supplemental arm (not statistically significant).

- After adjustment for baseline ROP severity, plus disease, race, and gestational age, the odds ratio (supplemental vs. conventional) for progression was 0.72.

- Mean progression time to threshold disease was 2.4 weeks for eyes in the conventional arm and 2.7 weeks for eyes in the supplemental arm.

- Eyes with plus disease at study entry progressed to threshold disease most rapidly, at a mean of 1.6 and 2.2 weeks in the conventional arm and supplemental arm, respectively.

- Final structural status of all study eyes at 3 months of corrected age showed similar rates of severe sequelae in both treatment arms.

- Retinal detachments or folds: 4.4% conventional vs. 4.1% supplemental.

- Macular ectopia: 3.9% conventional vs. 3.9% supplemental.

- Pneumonia and/or exacerbations of chronic lung disease occurred in more infants in the supplemental arm (8.5% conventional vs. 13.2% supplemental).

- At 50 weeks PMA, fewer conventional than supplemental infants remained hospitalized (6.8% vs. 12.7%, $P = .01$), on oxygen (37.0% vs. 46.8%, $P = .02$), and on diuretics (24.4% vs. 35.8%, $P = .002$).

- Growth and developmental milestones did not differ between the 2 arms.

Criticisms and Limitations: The STOP-ROP study examined the effects of oxygen supplementation *after* diagnosis of prethreshold ROP and therefore cannot be used to make assumptions about oxygen supplementation before this development, that is, there are no data to suggest that higher oxygen saturation levels are safe for the early immature eye that does not yet have established ROP.

The STOP-ROP study does not rule out a potential small reduction in the rate of ROP progression with supplemental oxygen, and a subgroup analysis suggests that supplemental oxygen, as used in this study, may be more effective in prethreshold ROP without plus disease.

Other Relevant Studies and Information:

- The HOPE-ROP Trial was a randomized, controlled clinical trial to determine the rate of progression from prethreshold to threshold retinopathy of prematurity (ROP) in infants excluded from STOP-ROP because their median arterial oxygen saturation by pulse oximetry (SpO2) values were >94% in room air at the time of prethreshold diagnosis, and to compare them with infants who were enrolled in STOP-ROP and had median SpO2 <94% in room air.[2] The HOPE-ROP cohort were of a higher gestational age (26.2 weeks vs. 25.2 weeks) and higher PMA at time of prethreshold ROP diagnosis (36.7 weeks vs. 35.4 weeks). HOPE-ROP infants progressed to threshold ROP 25% of the time compared with 46% of STOP-ROP infants. After gestational age, race, PMA at prethreshold diagnosis, zone 1 disease, and plus disease at prethreshold diagnosis were controlled for, logistic regression analysis showed that HOPE-ROP infants progressed from prethreshold to threshold ROP less often than STOP-ROP infants (odds ratio: 0.61).

- ROP is a complex, multifactorial disease. Oxygen is a key mediator, but the exact pathophysiology is not yet understood, and the best oxygen profiles to reduce ROP risk while optimizing preterm infant health and development remain unknown.[3,4]

  - A retrospective cohort study of premature infants undergoing ROP screening before and after implementation of an oxygen therapy protocol to inhibit further progression of ROP found that progression from stage 2 to stage 3 ROP in premature infants was significantly decreased after implementation of the protocol, without a corresponding increase in pulmonary morbidity.[5]

    - 44% of infants without the oxygen therapy protocol progressed beyond stage 2, compared to 23% of infants after protocol implementation ($P = .001$).

Summary and Implications: The STOP-ROP data clearly demonstrated that oxygen at saturation levels of 96% to 99% does not increase the severity of ROP in the eyes of infants with prethreshold or less than prethreshold ROP. If an infant requires saturations of 96% to 99% for cardiopulmonary reasons, fear about causing worse ROP is not a reason to withhold the oxygen. However, the risk of adverse pulmonary events is increased.

CLINICAL CASE: A PREMATURE INFANT WITH PRETHRESHOLD ROP IN ONE EYE

Case History

Ophthalmological exam of a premature infant reveals that the infant has prethreshold ROP in one eye. Your assistant notes that pulse oximetry readings average around 90%–92% in room air. She suggests using supplemental oxygen to bring the pulse oximeter readings closer to 99% to possibly prevent progression to threshold disease. Based on the results of the STOP-ROP trial, what is the likely outcome of using supplemental oxygen in this infant?

A. No change in retinal or general health.
B. Significant increase in progression to threshold disease.
C. Significant decrease in progression to threshold disease.
D. No significant effect and possibility of increased respiratory complications.

Suggested Answer

Option D is correct. The STOP-ROP study showed that use of supplemental oxygen at pulse oximetry saturations of 96%–99% did not cause additional progression of prethreshold ROP but also did not significantly reduce the number of infants requiring peripheral ablative surgery. The study did show that supplemental oxygen increased the risk of adverse pulmonary events including pneumonia and/or exacerbations of chronic lung disease and the need for oxygen, diuretics, and hospitalization at 3 months of corrected age.

References

1. Supplemental Therapeutic Oxygen for Prethreshold Retinopathy Of Prematurity (STOP-ROP), a randomized, controlled trial. I: Primary outcomes. *Pediatrics.* 2000;105(2):295–310.
2. McGregor ML, Bremer DL, Cole C, et al.; HOPE-ROP Multicenter Group. High Oxygen Percentage in Retinopathy of Prematurity study. Retinopathy of prematurity outcome in infants with prethreshold retinopathy of prematurity and oxygen saturation >94% in room air: the high oxygen percentage in retinopathy of prematurity study. *Pediatrics.* 2002;110(3):540–4.
3. Hartnett ME, Lane RH. Effects of oxygen on the development and severity of retinopathy of prematurity. *J AAPOS.* 2013;17(3):229–34.
4. Owen LA, Hartnett ME. Current concepts of oxygen management in retinopathy of prematurity. *J Ophthalmic Vis Res.* 2014;9(1):94–100.
5. Colaizy TT, Longmuir S, Gertsch K, Abràmoff MD, Klein JM. Use of a supplemental oxygen protocol to suppress progression of retinopathy of prematurity. *Invest Ophthalmol Vis Sci.* 2017;58(2):887–91.

27

Early Treatment of Prethreshold Retinopathy of Prematurity*

Early Treatment for Retinopathy of Prematurity (ETROP) Study

> Early treatment of high-risk prethreshold ROP significantly reduced unfavorable outcomes in both primary and secondary (structural) measures.
> —ETROP Cooperative Group[1]

Research Question: In infants with unilateral or bilateral high-risk retinopathy of prematurity (ROP), does peripheral retinal ablation reduce unfavorable outcomes, compared to conventional management (observation and treatment if the eye develops threshold ROP)?[1]

Funding: National Eye Institute, National Institutes of Health.

Year Study Began: 2001.

Year Study Published: 2004.

Study Location: 26 centers in the United States.

---

* Basic and Clinical Science Course, Section 6. *Pediatric Ophthalmology and Strabismus.* San Francisco: American Academy of Ophthalmology; 2018–2019: 326, 332.

* Basic and Clinical Science Course, Section 12. *Retina and Vitreous.* San Francisco: American Academy of Ophthalmology; 2018–2019: 178, 185.

Who Was Studied: Infants who weighed less than 1251 g at birth with prethreshold ROP (defined as any Zone I ROP; or Zone II stage 2 with plus disease, or Zone II stage 3 without plus disease; or Zone II with less than 5 contiguous or 8 cumulative clock hours of stage 3 ROP with plus disease) and a risk of progression to an unfavorable outcome in the absence of treatment ≥15%, calculated using a risk analysis model developed using longitudinal natural history data obtained from the Cryotherapy for Retinopathy of Prematurity (CRYO-ROP) study.[2]

Who Was Excluded: Infants in whom either eye had developed threshold ROP prior to randomization were excluded from the study.

How Many Patients: 401.

Study Overview: Early Treatment for Retinopathy of Prematurity (ETROP) was a randomized, controlled, clinical trial (Figure 27.1).[1,3-5]

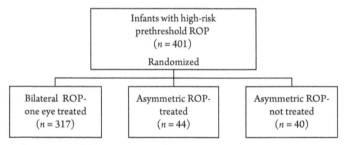

Figure 27.1 Summary of the ETROP trial.

Study Intervention: Infants with bilateral high-risk prethreshold ROP had 1 eye randomized to early retinal ablative treatment (within 48 hours of diagnosis) and the fellow eye (control eye) managed conventionally—that is, observation and treatment if the eye developed threshold ROP. In asymmetric cases, the eye with high-risk prethreshold ROP was randomized to early retinal ablative treatment or to conventional management. Peripheral retinal ablation was generally laser therapy, but cryotherapy was allowed.

Follow-Up: 6 and 9 months.

Endpoints: The primary outcome was monocular grating acuity assessed by masked testers using the Teller acuity card procedure at 9 months corrected age. The visual acuity outcome was divided into four categories of functional response, and these functional outcome categories were further grouped into "favorable" and "unfavorable" designations. Structural examinations were performed at 6 and

9 months. At 6 months, an unfavorable outcome was defined as (1) a posterior retinal fold involving the macula, (2) a retinal detachment involving the macula, or (3) retrolental tissue or "mass" obscuring the view of the posterior pole. At the 9-month examination, eyes that had received a vitrectomy or scleral buckle were classified for study purposes as having an unfavorable structural outcome.

RESULTS

- The mean birth weight was 703 g and the mean gestational age was 25.3 weeks. At the time of randomization, 79.1% of the infants had high-risk prethreshold disease bilaterally. The remaining 20.9% of infants had asymmetric disease, with high-risk prethreshold ROP in only one eye.
- The average age at the time of high-risk prethreshold treatment was 35.2 weeks postmenstrual age and 10.0 weeks chronological age. The average age for treatment of eyes in the conventionally managed group that went on to threshold was 37.0 weeks postmenstrual age and 11.9 weeks chronological age.
- Grating acuity results (average corrected age [age from expected date of delivery] 10.3 months at the time of assessment) showed a reduction in unfavorable visual acuity outcomes with earlier treatment, from 19.8% to 14.3% ($P < .005$).
- Unfavorable structural outcomes (average corrected age 9.8 months at the time of assessment) were reduced from 15.6% to 9.0% ($P < .001$).
  - Among the 30 high-risk prethreshold treated eyes that had an unfavorable structural outcome at 9 months, two had a partial retinal detachment involving the macula, 23 had undergone a vitrectomy or a scleral buckle, and five had total retinal detachment. Among the 51 conventionally managed eyes with an unfavorable outcome, four had a partial retinal detachment involving the macula, 43 had undergone a vitrectomy or a scleral buckle, and four had total retinal detachment.
  - Structural outcome results at the 6-month examination were similar to those at 9 months.
- The distribution of refractive errors at the 9-month examination was similar between the high-risk prethreshold treated eyes that received early treatment and those that were conventionally managed.
- Cataract/aphakia that was not associated with total retinal detachment or vitrectomy was found in four eyes (1.2%) in the group treated at high-risk prethreshold and in four eyes (1.2%) in the conventionally managed group.
- Ocular complication rates were similar in the 2 groups.

- Systemic complications (including apnea, bradycardia, and reintubation)
  were higher following treatment at high-risk prethreshold, probably
  because of the younger average postmenstrual age at which the treatment
  of high-risk prethreshold eyes occurred (35.2 weeks vs. 37.0 weeks).

Criticisms and Limitations: The possible adverse effects and trade-offs related
to earlier treatment include an increased rate of systemic complications, potential long-term risks of earlier treatment, an increase in the number of eye
examinations needed to detect prethreshold ROP, and an increased frequency of
treatment of eyes that would otherwise have undergone spontaneous regression
of ROP.

Other Relevant Studies and Information:

- Further follow-up of 339 of 374 (90.6%) surviving children of ETROP
  showed that at 2 years of age, unfavorable structural outcomes were
  reduced from 15.4% in conventionally managed eyes to 9.1% in earlier-
  treated eyes ($P = .002$). Ophthalmic side effects (excluding retinal
  structure) from the ROP or its treatment were similar in the earlier-
  treated eyes and the conventionally managed eyes.[6]
- At 6 years of age, there was no statistically significant benefit for
  early treatment (24.3% vs. 28.6% [corrected] unfavorable outcome;
  $P = .15$). Analysis of 6-year visual acuity results according to the Type
  1 and 2 clinical algorithm showed a benefit for Type 1 eyes (25.1% vs.
  32.8%; $P = .02$) treated early but not Type 2 eyes (23.6% vs. 19.4%;
  $P = .37$). Early-treated eyes showed a significantly better structural
  outcome compared with conventionally managed eyes (8.9% vs.
  15.2% unfavorable outcome; $P < .001$), with no greater risk of ocular
  complications.[7]

Summary and Implications: The results of this study showed that it is possible
to identify characteristics of ROP that predict which eyes are most likely to benefit from early peripheral retinal ablation. A clinical algorithm was developed to
discriminate between eyes with prethreshold ROP that are at highest risk for retinal detachment and blindness and eyes with prethreshold ROP likely to show
spontaneous regression of ROP. The use of this algorithm circumvents the need
for computer-based calculation of low risk or high risk, as was used in this study.
The algorithm does not take into account all of the other known risk factors (e.g.,

extent of stage 3, birth weight, etc.), and therefore some clinical judgment is required.

Peripheral retinal ablation should be considered for any eye with:

Type I ROP

- Zone I, any stage ROP with plus disease, or
- Zone I, stage 3, with or without plus disease, or
- Zone II, stage 2 or 3 ROP, with plus disease

NOTE: Plus disease, in this algorithm, requires at least two quadrants (usually 6 or more clock hours) of dilation and tortuosity of the posterior retinal blood vessels and, hence, the presence of significant disease.

Observation with serial eye examinations should be considered for any eye with:

Type II ROP

- Zone I, stage 1 or 2 with no plus disease, or
- Zone II, stage 3 with no plus disease

Treatment should be considered for an eye with type II ROP when progression to type I status or threshold ROP occurs.

CLINICAL CASE: A PREMATURE INFANT WITH PRETHRESHOLD ROP

Case History

A female infant was born at 26 weeks gestation with a birth weight of 950 g. Assisted ventilation was immediately started with 100% oxygen and continued for three weeks with a FiO2 (fraction inspiratory oxygen) of 25%. The partial pressure of oxygen (PO2) was maintained at 50–70 mm Hg, but there were three short episodes of PO2 above 100 mm Hg. Examination performed at 4 weeks revealed that the right eye had stage 3 ROP in Zone 1 from 1 o'clock to 6 o'clock with no congestion of vessels. The left eye had severe active ROP (stage III) in zone II, 360 degrees. There was no congestion of vessels. What do you recommend to the parents as the best treatment option for her according to the clinical algorithm based on the ETROP trial?

A. Repeat examination of both eyes in 1 week.
B. Retinal ablation of right eye, observation and serial examinations of the left eye.
C. Retinal ablation of left eye, observation and serial examinations of the right eye.
D. Retinal ablation of both eyes.

Suggested Answer

According to the algorithm based on the ETROP study the right eye has Type I ROP and needs peripheral retinal ablation whereas the left eye has Type II ROP and requires serial examinations (option B).

References

1. Good WV; Early Treatment for Retinopathy of Prematurity Cooperative Group. Final results of the Early Treatment for Retinopathy of Prematurity (ETROP) randomized trial. *Trans Am Ophthalmol Soc.* 2004;102:233–48; discussion 248–50.
2. Hardy RJ, Palmer EA, Dobson V, et al.; Cryotherapy for Retinopathy of Prematurity Cooperative Group. Risk analysis of prethreshold retinopathy of prematurity. *Arch Ophthalmol.* 2003;121(12):1697–701.
3. Good WV, Hardy RJ. The multicenter study of early treatment for retinopathy of prematurity (ETROP). *Ophthalmology.* 2001;108(6):1013–4.
4. Early Treatment for Retinopathy of Prematurity Cooperative Group. Multicenter trial of early treatment for retinopathy of prematurity: study design. *Contr Clin Trials.* 2004;25(3):311–25.
5. Early Treatment For Retinopathy Of Prematurity Cooperative Group. Revised indications for the treatment of retinopathy of prematurity: results of the early treatment for retinopathy of prematurity randomized trial. *Arch Ophthalmol.* 2003;121(12):1684–94.
6. The Early Treatment for Retinopathy of Prematurity Cooperative Group. The Early Treatment for Retinopathy Of Prematurity Study: structural findings at age 2 years. *Br J Ophthalmol.* 2006;90(11):1378–82.
7. Early Treatment for Retinopathy of Prematurity Cooperative Group, Good WV, Hardy RJ, Dobson V, et al. Final visual acuity results in the early treatment for retinopathy of prematurity study. *Arch Ophthalmol.* 2010;128(6):663–71.

Intravitreal Bevacizumab for Stage 3+ Retinopathy of Prematurity*

Bevacizumab Eliminates the Angiogenic Threat of Retinopathy of Prematurity (BEAT-ROP) Study

Intravitreal bevacizumab monotherapy, as compared with conventional laser therapy, in infants with stage 3+ retinopathy of prematurity showed a significant benefit for zone I but not zone II disease. Development of peripheral retinal vessels continued after treatment with intravitreal bevacizumab, but conventional laser therapy led to permanent destruction of the peripheral retina.

—BEAT-ROP COOPERATIVE GROUP[1]

Research Question: Is intravitreal bevacizumab (IVB) monotherapy an effective therapy for treating zone I or zone II posterior stage 3+ (stage 3 with plus disease) retinopathy of prematurity (ROP)?[1]

Funding: Research to Prevent Blindness (New York, NY); National Eye Institute, National Institutes of Health; Hermann Eye Fund (Houston, TX); Alfred W. Lasher III Professorship (Houston, TX); University of Texas Health Science Center at Houston-Center for Clinical Translational Science-Clinical Research Center (Houston, TX).

---

* Basic and Clinical Science Course, Section 12. *Retina and Vitreous*. San Francisco: American Academy of Ophthalmology; 2018–2019: 186–187.

Year Study Began: 2008.

Year Study Published: 2011.

Study Location: 15 hospitals in the United States.

Who Was Studied: Newborns with birth weight of 1500 g or less and a gestational age of 30 weeks or less who had zone I or zone II posterior stage 3+ (i.e., stage 3 with plus disease) ROP.

Who Was Excluded: Infants with stage 4 or 5 ROP in either eye.

How Many Patients: 150.

Study Overview: BEAT-ROP was a prospective, randomized, controlled trial (Figure 28.1).[1]

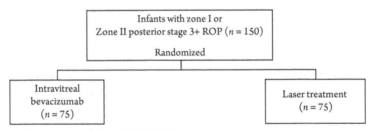

Figure 28.1 Summary of the BEAT-ROP study.

Study Intervention: Sixty-seven infants had zone I ROP: 34 were randomly assigned to IVB therapy (0.625 mg in 0.025 ml) and 34 to conventional laser treatment. Eighty-three infants had zone II posterior ROP: 42 were randomly assigned to IVB therapy and 41 to conventional laser treatment. Serial eye examinations began at 4 weeks' chronologic age or 31 weeks' postmenstrual age, whichever was later. In all groups, the mean gestational age at study entry was 24 weeks; the mean postmenstrual age at the time of treatment was approximately 34–36 weeks.

Follow-Up: 54 weeks.

Endpoints: Recurrence of ROP (documented by RetCam photography) in one or both eyes requiring retreatment before 54 weeks postmenstrual age.

RESULTS

- The rate of recurrence of ROP for zone I and posterior zone II combined was significantly higher with conventional laser therapy (26%) than with IVB (6%) ($P = .002$).
  - The absolute difference between the two groups in the risk of recurrence was 20 percentage points.
- The rate of recurrence with zone I disease alone was significantly higher with conventional laser therapy (42%) than with IVB (6%) ($P = .003$).
  - Recurrence after IVB occurred in two eyes (unilateral), with macular dragging in one of the two eyes.
  - Recurrence after conventional laser therapy occurred in 23 eyes (5 unilateral and 9 bilateral), with macular dragging in 16 eyes and retinal detachment in 2 eyes.
- The rate of recurrence with zone II posterior disease alone did not differ significantly between the laser-therapy group (12%) and the bevacizumab group (5%) ($P = .27$).
  - Retinopathy recurred in four eyes (bilateral in two infants) after IVB therapy, with no instances of macular dragging but with retinal detachment in two eyes (bilateral).
  - After conventional laser therapy, retinopathy recurred in nine eyes (one unilateral and four bilateral), with macular dragging in six eyes but with no instances of retinal detachment.
- ROP recurred in 2 of 62 eyes in infants with zone I disease and in 4 of 78 eyes in infants with zone II posterior disease. For both zones considered together, the mean time to recurrence was 16.0 weeks, compared to 6.2 weeks for 32 eyes after conventional laser therapy.
- Seven infants (5 who underwent IVB therapy and 2 who underwent conventional laser therapy) died before 54 weeks' postmenstrual age and without having reached the primary outcome.

Criticisms and Limitations: Overall, 57% of the infants were Hispanic. Anecdotally, Hispanic infants have been more difficult to treat.[2] Whether other racial/ethnic groups would show the same results is not known.

The study was not large enough to determine possible systemic or local toxic effects of bevacizumab. The long-term safety of bevacizumab could also not be determined.

Additional research is needed to determine the dose of IVB that should be used for retinopathy of prematurity at any stage versus advanced disease and for standard (type 1) versus aggressive posterior (type 2) disease.

Other Relevant Studies and Information:

- A randomized, multicenter clinical trial found that the use of pegaptanib with laser therapy was efficacious in 91.2% compared with 69.0% in controls. The use of bevacizumab monotherapy was efficacious in 95.7% compared with 78.1% in controls.[3]
- A retrospective case series of premature infants with type 1 ROP (subdivided into stage 3+ ROP and aggressive posterior ROP [APROP]) in zone I or zone II posterior who received intravitreal bevacizumab (IVB) monotherapy and were followed up for at least 65 weeks adjusted age found that the incidence of recurrence was 8.3% for infants and 7.2% for eyes. The recurrence risk period was between approximately 45 and 55 weeks adjusted age for 90.0% of infants and 94.1% of eyes, with mean recurrence of 51.2 weeks adjusted age and mean interval of 16.2 weeks between treatments.[4]
- A Cochrane review (6 trials, 383 infants) of the efficacy and safety of anti–vascular endothelial growth factor (VEGF) drugs when used either as monotherapy or in combination with planned cryo/laser therapy in preterm infants with type 1 ROP (defined as zone I any stage with plus disease, zone I stage 3 with or without plus disease, or zone II stage 2 or 3 with plus disease) concluded: "The quality of the evidence was very low to low for most outcomes due to risk of detection bias and other biases. . . . Further studies are needed to evaluate the effect of anti-VEGF agents on structural and functional outcomes in childhood and delayed systemic effects including adverse neurodevelopmental outcomes."[5]
  - IVB, when used as monotherapy, reduces the risk of refractive errors during childhood but does not reduce the risk of retinal detachment or recurrence of ROP in infants with type 1 ROP. While the intervention might reduce the risk of recurrence of ROP in infants with zone I ROP, it can potentially result in higher risk of recurrence requiring retreatment in those with zone II ROP.
  - Intravitreal pegaptanib, when used in conjunction with laser therapy, reduces the risk of retinal detachment as well as the recurrence of ROP in infants with type 1 ROP.
- A randomized clinical trial to compare the efficacy of IVB injection with conventional laser photocoagulation in eyes with type 1 zone II

retinopathy of prematurity (ROP) found that both IVB injection and laser photocoagulation were effective methods for the treatment of type 1 zone II ROP.[6] However, retreatment requirement may be higher in the IVB injection group. IVB reinjection is an effective option for retreatment in persistent cases.

Summary and Implications: This study demonstrated the increased efficacy of IVB as compared with conventional laser therapy for stage 3+ ROP in zone I in infants up to 54 weeks' postmenstrual age. Intravitreal bevacizumab does not permanently destroy retinal tissue and allows for continued vessel growth into the peripheral retina; recurrence of ROP can still occur, indicating the need for continued close follow-up.

CLINICAL CASE: A PREMATURE INFANT WITH BILATERAL ROP

Case History
You evaluate a 30-week old preterm baby in the neonatal ICU. On exam you note stage 3 Zone I ROP in the right eye and stage 3 Zone II ROP in the left eye. How would you proceed with counseling the parents concerning treatment options?

A. Both eyes will benefit more from panretinal photocoagulation (PRP) than bevacizumab.
B. The right eye will benefit from either PRP or bevacizumab equally, but the left eye may benefit more from bevacizumab.
C. The right eye may benefit more from bevacizumab but the right eye will benefit from either PRP or bevacizumab equally.
D. Both eyes will benefit more from bevacizumab than PRP.

Suggested Answer
Option C. The results of the BEAT-ROP trial suggest that bevacizumab is more efficacious in Stage 3 Zone I disease than monotherapy with PRP. However, with Zone II disease the effects were equivocal between the two therapy modalities.

References

1. Mintz-Hittner HA, Kennedy KA, Chuang AZ; BEAT-ROP Cooperative Group. Efficacy of intravitreal bevacizumab for stage 3+ retinopathy of prematurity. *N Engl J Med.* 2011;364(7):603–15.
2. Stuart, Annie. Current ROP therapies: how laser and Anti-VEGF compare. *EyeNet Magazine.* Feb 2014. https://www.aao.org/eyenet/article/current-rop-therapies-how-laser-antivegf-compare.
3. Mintz-Hittner HA. Intravitreal pegaptanib as adjunctive treatment for stage 3+ ROP shown to be effective in a prospective, randomized, controlled multicenter clinical trial. *Eur J Ophthalmol.* 2012;22(5):685–6.
4. Mintz-Hittner HA, Geloneck MM, Chuang AZ. Clinical management of recurrent retinopathy of prematurity after intravitreal bevacizumab monotherapy. *Ophthalmology.* 2016;123(9):1845–55.
5. Sankar MJ, Sankar J, Chandra P. Anti-vascular endothelial growth factor (VEGF) drugs for treatment of retinopathy of prematurity. *Cochrane Database Syst Rev.* 2018;1:CD009734.
6. Roohipoor R, Torabi H, Karkhaneh R, Riazi-Eafahani M. Comparison of intravitreal bevacizumab injection and laser photocoagulation for type 1 zone II retinopathy of prematurity. *J Curr Ophthalmol.* 2018;31(1):61–65.

29

Photocoagulation for Diabetic Macular Edema

Early Treatment Diabetic Retinopathy Study (ETDRS) Report Number 1 *

Focal photocoagulation of "clinically significant" diabetic macular edema substantially reduces the risk of visual loss. Focal treatment also increases the chance of visual improvement, decreases the frequency of persistent macular edema, and causes only minor visual field losses.

—ETDRS RESEARCH GROUP[1]

Research Question: Is photocoagulation effective in the treatment of diabetic macular edema (DME)?[1]

Funding: National Eye Institute, National Institutes of Health.

Year Study Began: 1980.

Year Study Published: 1985.

Study Location: 29 centers in the United States.

Who Was Studied: Diabetic patients with mild to moderate nonproliferative diabetic retinopathy and macular edema in one or both eyes. Macular edema was defined as retinal thickening at or within 1 disc diameter of the center of

---

* Basic and Clinical Science Course, Section 12. *Retina and Vitreous.* San Francisco: American Academy of Ophthalmology; 2018–2019: 110, 114–115.

the macula or definite hard exudates in this region. Macular edema was designated as being "clinically significant" if at least one of these characteristics was present on stereo contact lens biomicroscopy and photography: thickening of the retina at or within 500 microns of the center of the macula; hard exudates at or within 500 microns of the center of the macula, if associated with thickening of adjacent retina (not residual hard exudates remaining after disappearance of retinal thickening); a zone or zones of retinal thickening 1 disc area or larger, any part of which is within 1 disc diameter of the center of the macula.

Who Was Excluded: Patients with "high-risk" proliferative retinopathy (moderate or severe optic nerve neovascularization or any neovascularization with hemorrhage), other significant ocular disease, or visual acuity worse than 20/200 were ineligible.

How Many Patients: 1,876.

Study Overview: The ETDRS was a prospective, randomized clinical trial (Figure 29.1).[1,2]

Nearly 4,000 diabetic patients with early proliferative retinopathy, moderate to severe nonproliferative retinopathy, and/or DME in each eye were enrolled. This paper reports the findings in the subgroup of eyes in the ETDRS that were identified as having mild to moderate nonproliferative diabetic retinopathy and macular edema.

Study Intervention: Eyes were randomly assigned to immediate photocoagulation or deferral of photocoagulation until high-risk proliferative retinopathy developed. The eyes assigned to immediate photocoagulation were then randomly divided into two photocoagulation regimens: one half of the eyes received only focal treatment for macular edema initially. This report compares these focally treated eyes with those randomized to deferral of photocoagulation.

Discrete lesions (microaneurysms and other sites of focal leakage) were treated with focal photocoagulation (50–100 micron argon blue-green or green-only burns) if they were located within 2 disc diameters of the center of the macula but at least 500 microns from the center. (If vision was less than 20/40 and the retinal edema and leakage persisted, treatment of lesions up to 300 microns from the center was recommended, unless there was perifoveal capillary dropout.) Areas of diffuse leakage or nonperfusion within 2 disc diameters of the center of the macula were treated in a grid pattern. Follow-up focal photocoagulation was

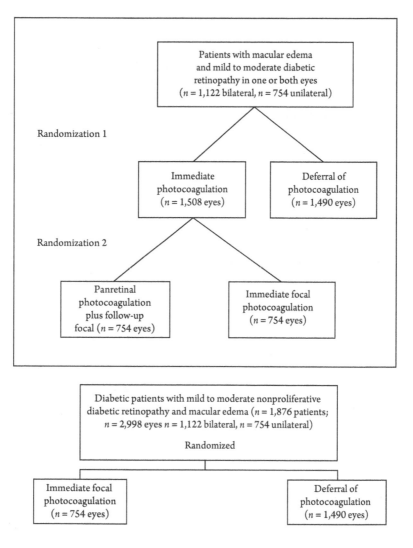

Figure 29.1. Summary of the ETDRS.

required for all eyes assigned to immediate treatment that had persistent clinically significant macular edema and treatable lesions.

Follow-Up: 12 months (for 80% of the patients); 36 months (for 35% of the patients).

Endpoints: Change in visual acuity, specifically a loss of 15 or more letters, equivalent to a three-line visual acuity decrease on the ETDRS chart or a doubling of the visual angle (e.g., 20/20 to 20/40 or 20/100 to 20/200).

RESULTS

- Eyes assigned to immediate focal photocoagulation were about half as likely to lose 15 or more letters on the ETDRS eye chart compared with eyes assigned to deferral of photocoagulation: 5% vs. 8% at one year ($P < .01$), 7% vs. 16% at two years ($P < .001$), and 12% vs. 24% at three years ($P < .001$).
  - Differences between the groups in the percentages of eyes with visual acuity worse than 20/100) at each time point showed the same pattern.
- In eyes with a pretreatment visual acuity of 20/40 or worse, an improvement in visual acuity of six or more letters (more than one line on the ETDRS visual acuity chart) was much more frequent in treated eyes than in eyes assigned to deferral of treatment.
- There was clear beneficial effect of immediate focal treatment in eyes with clinically significant macular edema; in those eyes, the differences in rates of visual loss between the immediate focal photocoagulation and deferral of photocoagulation groups were statistically significant at the 8-month follow-up visit and thereafter.
  - Eyes in which macular edema was not clinically significant at baseline had low rates of visual loss, especially during the first year of follow-up, in both the immediate and deferral of photocoagulation groups.
- At 1 year 35% of eyes with retinal thickening that were assigned to immediate focal treatment had persistent retinal thickening with the center of the macula involved compared with 63% of eyes assigned to deferred photocoagulation.
- Very few adverse effects of focal photocoagulation were observed—only minor adverse effects on central visual fields and no adverse effects on color vision.

Criticisms and Limitations: It was not possible to determine the effects of focal treatment in the absence of panretinal photocoagulation for this group. It was also not possible to determine whether argon green laser was better than argon blue-green photocoagulation.

Optical coherence tomography (OCT), not available at the time of the ETDRS, is used now to assess the severity of macular edema. Using OCT, "clinically significant" macular edema is now classified into center-involved DME (CI-DME) and non-center-involved DME (NCI-DME). A modified focal/grid laser treatment is now preferred.

Other Relevant Studies and Information:

- Intravitreal injections of anti–vascular endothelial growth factors (VEGFs) and steroids are increasingly used and recommended for initial and follow-up management of macular edema; however, laser photocoagulation treatment continues to have an important role. Ranibizumab has been shown to be superior to laser in macular edema treatment, providing excellent long-term visual outcomes; frequent injections may be necessary to properly control DME and maximize the visual benefits. Macular laser therapy may still play an important role as an adjuvant treatment because it is able to improve macular thickness outcomes and reduce the number of injections needed. See [3-5] for reviews of recent and ongoing trials of intravitreal injections in combination with prompt or deferred laser treatment.
- Protocol I was a multicenter randomized clinical trial comparing the visual outcomes of patients treated with 0.5 mg intravitreal ranibizumab with either prompt or deferred (by 24 weeks) laser, 4 mg intravitreal triamcinolone with prompt laser, or sham injection with prompt laser for the treatment of CI DME. A total of 854 adult patients with type 1 or 2 diabetes and any level of nonproliferative diabetic retinopathy or proliferative retinopathy with adequate panretinal photocoagulation, with best corrected visual acuity 20/32 to 20/320 (Snellen equivalent) and visual loss attributed to macular edema, or retinal thickening with central subfield thickness of at least 250 μm by OCT.[6] The main findings were:
  - Intravitreal ranibizumab treatment provides superior visual outcomes compared to conventional laser treatment.
  - Adjunctive laser treatment does not appear to provide substantial visual benefit compared to ranibizumab treatment alone, but may reduce the number of injections required to resolve macular edema. Deferral of laser is likely beneficial in patients with worse initial visual acuity.
  - Delayed initiation of intravitreal ranibizumab therapy provides improved visual outcome among patients initially treated with conventional laser photocoagulation or triamcinolone, but the magnitude of the benefit is not as great as is observed when ranibizumab treatment is initiated promptly.
  - The number of ranibizumab injections required to achieve the desired visual outcome decreases substantially after the first year, with the majority of patients not requiring further treatment after 3 years.

- Patients who do not have a rapid response to ranibizumab still display long-term benefit to continued therapy, although perhaps less than those with immediate improvement.
- Intravitreal ranibizumab is not only effective in reducing retinal edema and improving BCVA among patients with macular edema, it is also a disease modifying therapy and induces improvement of the diabetic retinopathy severity score by 2 or more steps in approximately one third of patients.

Summary and Implications: Focal argon laser photocoagulation is recommended for all eyes with clinically significant macular edema and mild or moderate nonproliferative diabetic retinopathy, regardless of the level of visual acuity. Focal photocoagulation should also be considered for all eyes with clinically significant macular edema and more severe nonproliferative or proliferative retinopathy. Patients should be followed up frequently to determine whether additional treatment is needed for the persistence or recrudescence of clinically significant macular edema.

CLINICAL CASE: A MAN WITH MILD NONPROLIFERATIVE DIABETIC RETINOPATHY AND MACULAR EDEMA

Case History

A 47-year-old man with a history of poorly controlled type 2 diabetes presents for a diabetic eye exam. The patient's vision is 20/25 in the right eye and 20/30 in the left eye. On dilated fundus exam he is found to have mild nonproliferative diabetic retinopathy in the mid-periphery in both eyes. On posterior pole examination he has thickening of the retina within 500 microns of the center of the macula in the right eye and hard exudates within 500 microns of the macula center and associated thickening of the adjacent retina in the left eye. In the absence of availability of ANY intraocular injections for treatment, what is your treatment recommendation based on findings from the ETDRS Report 1?

A. Observation until either severe NPDR or PDR develops in one eye.
B. Focal argon laser photocoagulation in both eyes.
C. Observation until vision decreases to < 20/40 in one eye, then focal argon laser photocoagulation in that eye.
D. Pan retinal photocoagulation in both eyes to treat prophylactically.

Suggested Answer

The patient has clinically significant macular edema and mild nonproliferative diabetic retinopathy, therefore, according to the ETDRS, focal argon laser photocoagulation is recommended (option B).

References

1. Photocoagulation for diabetic macular edema. Early Treatment Diabetic Retinopathy Study report number 1. Early Treatment Diabetic Retinopathy Study research group. *Arch Ophthalmol.* 1985;103(12):1796–806.
2. Early Treatment Diabetic Retinopathy Study design and baseline patient characteristics. ETDRS report number 7. *Ophthalmology.* 1991;98(5 Suppl):741–56.
3. Relhan N, Flynn HW Jr. The Early Treatment Diabetic Retinopathy Study historical review and relevance to today's management of diabetic macular edema. *Curr Opin Ophthalmol.* 2017;28(3):205–12.
4. Distefano LN, Garcia-Arumi J, Martinez-Castillo V, Boixadera A. Combination of anti-VEGF and laser photocoagulation for diabetic macular edema: a review. *J Ophthalmol.* 2017;2017:2407037.
5. Zucchiatti I, Bandello F. Intravitreal ranibizumab in diabetic macular edema: long-term outcomes. *Dev Ophthalmol.* 2017;60:63–70.
6. Mukkamala L, Bhagat N, Zarbin MA. Practical lessons from protocol I for the management of diabetic macular edema. *Dev Ophthalmol.* 2017;60:91–108.

30

Early Photocoagulation for Diabetic Retinopathy*

Early Treatment Diabetic Retinopathy Study (ETDRS) Report Number 9

Focal photocoagulation should be considered for eyes with clinically significant macular edema, preferably before scatter photocoagulation for high-risk proliferative retinopathy becomes urgent. Provided careful follow-up can be maintained, scatter photocoagulation is not recommended for eyes with mild or moderate non-proliferative diabetic retinopathy.

—ETDRS RESEARCH GROUP[1]

Research Questions:
1. When in the course of diabetic retinopathy is it most effective to initiate photocoagulation therapy?
2. Is photocoagulation effective in the treatment of macular edema?[1]

Funding: National Eye Institute, National Institutes of Health.

Year Study Began: 1980.

* Basic and Clinical Science Course, Section 12. *Retina and Vitreous*. San Francisco: American Academy of Ophthalmology; 2018–2019: 99–101.

Year Study Published: 1991.

Study Location: 29 centers in the United States.

Who Was Studied: Diabetic patients, between 18 and 70 years of age, with, in both eyes: (1) no macular edema, visual acuity of 20/40 or better, and moderate or severe nonproliferative diabetic retinopathy or early proliferative diabetic retinopathy, or (2) macular edema, visual acuity of 20/200 or better, and mild, moderate, or severe nonproliferative diabetic retinopathy or early proliferative diabetic retinopathy.

Who Was Excluded: Patients with "high-risk" proliferative retinopathy (moderate or severe optic nerve neovascularization or any neovascularization with hemorrhage), other significant ocular disease, or visual acuity worse than 20/200 were ineligible.

How Many Patients: 3,711.

Study Overview: The ETDRS was a prospective, randomized clinical trial (Figure 30.1).[1,2]

Study Intervention: Three groups were defined by the severity of retinopathy at baseline and the presence or absence of macular edema: (1) eyes without macular edema and moderate-to-severe nonproliferative or early proliferative retinopathy; (2) eyes with macular edema and mild-to-moderate nonproliferative retinopathy; (3) eyes with macular edema and severe nonproliferative or early proliferative retinopathy. Within each group, 1 eye of each patient was assigned randomly to early photocoagulation (scatter and/or focal) and the other eye to "deferral of photocoagulation." Eyes selected for early photocoagulation received 1 of 4 different combinations of scatter (panretinal) and focal treatment. Full scatter photocoagulation was initiated in eyes assigned to deferral as soon as high-risk proliferative retinopathy was detected. If clinically significant macular edema was present at that time, focal photocoagulation was initiated also, but only for those patients whose strategy for early photocoagulation for the fellow eye included delayed focal photocoagulation.

Follow-Up: 9 years.

Endpoints: The primary endpoint used to compare early photocoagulation with deferral of photocoagulation was the rate of development of "severe visual loss," defined as visual acuity less than 5/200 at two consecutive follow-up visits.

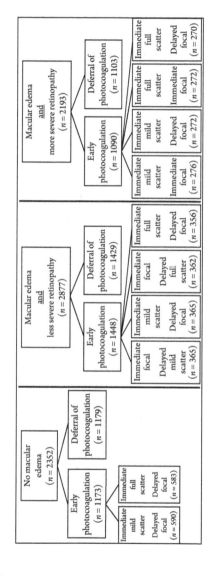

Figure 30.1 Summary of the ETDRS.

The primary endpoint for assessing the effects of photocoagulation on macular edema was the occurrence of "moderate visual loss," defined as loss of 15 or more letters (equivalent of 3 lines) between baseline and follow-up visit on the visual acuity charts used in the ETDRS.

RESULTS

- Early photocoagulation treatment, compared with deferral of photocoagulation, was associated with a small reduction in the incidence of severe visual loss (visual acuity less than 5/200 at two consecutive visits for at least 4 months), but 5-year rates were low in both the early treatment and deferral groups (2.6% and 3.7%, respectively).
- Compared with deferral of photocoagulation, early treatment did result in a marked reduction in the rate of developing high-risk proliferative diabetic retinopathy.
- Strategies for photocoagulation that included immediate full scatter photocoagulation reduced the rate of developing high-risk proliferative diabetic retinopathy by approximately 50%, while strategies that included immediate mild scatter reduced the rate by approximately 25%. Within all categories, the 5-year rate of developing high-risk proliferative diabetic retinopathy was highest in eyes assigned to deferral.
- Both the severity of retinopathy and the presence of macular edema at baseline were associated with the development of severe vision loss. However, the 5-year rate of severe vision loss, even among eyes with more severe retinopathy and macular edema, was only 6.5% in eyes assigned to deferral of photocoagulation.
- Immediate focal with delayed scatter photocoagulation (added only if more severe retinopathy developed) was the most effective strategy for eyes with macular edema and less severe retinopathy.
- Adverse effects of scatter photocoagulation on visual acuity and visual field were most evident in the months immediately following treatment and were less in eyes assigned to less extensive scatter photocoagulation. Therefore the benefits and risks of early photocoagulation must be considered. Early scatter photocoagulation is not recommended for eyes with mild to moderate retinopathy, but should be considered as retinopathy approaches the high risk stages.

Criticisms and Limitations: The ETDRS is regarded as a very good quality and detailed study. However, developments since the time of the ETDRS may have changed the balance of benefits and harms. For example, there have been improvements in diabetes care, with better control of blood glucose, blood pressure, and lipids. Laser technologies have advanced, with different regimens, better targeting, and a trend to "lighter" laser treatment with the aim of causing fewer adverse effects but retaining the same effectiveness. New drugs for macular edema have become available, particularly the anti–vascular endo-thelial growth factor (VEGF) agents, which may also affect retinopathy, and are being used in combination with laser photocoagulation. Finally, advances in imaging, such as optical coherence tomography (OCT), make detection of macular edema more reliable.[3]

Other Relevant Studies and Information:

- An earlier ETDRS report recommended focal photocoagulation for all eyes with clinically significant macular edema and mild or moderate nonproliferative diabetic retinopathy to reduce the risk of visual loss.[4] (See chapter 29.)
- The ETDRS also found that aspirin did not prevent the development of high-risk proliferative retinopathy and did not reduce the risk of visual loss, nor did it increase the risk of vitreous hemorrhage.[5]
- The ETDRS did not present separate results for moderate/severe nonproliferative diabetic retinopathy and early proliferative diabetic retinopathy. A systematic review of panretinal photocoagulation and other forms of laser treatment and drug therapies for severe nonproliferative diabetic retinopathy recommended a trial using newer laser technologies and modes of treatment to show conclusively the efficacy of early laser treatment before proliferative diabetic retinopathy has developed.[6] An economic modeling study concluded: "PRP administered at the severe NPDR stage is likely to be cost-effective compared with delaying photocoagulation until HR-PDR develops. However, given the limitations of the evidence, these results need to be interpreted with caution. A trial of early versus deferred laser therapy is needed to provide better data based on modern treatments."[7]

Summary and Implications: Provided careful follow-up can be maintained, panretinal scatter photocoagulation is not recommended for eyes with mild or moderate nonproliferative diabetic retinopathy. When retinopathy is more se-vere, panretinal scatter photocoagulation should be considered and usually should not be delayed if the eye has reached the high-risk proliferative stage.

Focal treatment should be considered for eyes with macular edema that involves or threatens the center of the macula, preferably before scatter photocoagulation for high-risk proliferative retinopathy becomes urgent. Focal photocoagulation reduces the risk of moderate visual loss, increases the chance of visual improvement, and decreases the frequency of persistent macular edema.

CLINICAL CASE: A MAN WITH SEVERE NONPROLIFERATIVE DIABETIC RETINOPATHY

Case History
A 47-year-old man with poorly controlled type 2 diabetes mellitus presents for a diabetic eye exam. The patient's vision is 20/25 in both eyes. The anterior segment examination is within normal limits. On dilated fundus examination, you see dot blot hemorrhages and/or microaneurysms in all quadrants in both eyes. You also detect soft exudates, venous beading, and intraretinal microvascular abnormalities in at least 2 quadrants in both eyes. There is no macular edema in either eye. You do not see any new vessels either on the optic discs or elsewhere. Based on the ETDRS Report Number 9, what treatment do you recommend for the patient?

A. Tight diabetic control and close observation of the retinal findings.
B. Focal argon laser photocoagulation in both eyes.
C. Panretinal scatter argon laser photocoagulation in both eyes.
D. Pars plana vitrectomy in worst eye/observation of other eye.

Suggested Answer
The patient has severe nonproliferative diabetic retinopathy in both eyes and is at high risk of developing proliferative diabetic retinopathy. Therefore, based on the findings of ETDRS 9, panretinal scatter photocoagulation is indicated for this patient (option C).

References
1. Early photocoagulation for diabetic retinopathy. ETDRS report number 9. Early Treatment Diabetic Retinopathy Study Research Group. *Ophthalmology*. 1991;98(5 Suppl):766–85.
2. Early Treatment Diabetic Retinopathy Study design and baseline patient characteristics. ETDRS report number 7. *Ophthalmology*. 1991;98(5 Suppl):741–56.

3. Chapter 2. The landmark trials: Diabetic Retinopathy Study and Early Treatment Diabetic Retinopathy Study. In: Royle P, Mistry H, Auguste P, et al. Pan-retinal photocoagulation and other forms of laser treatment and drug therapies for non-proliferative diabetic retinopathy: systematic review and economic evaluation. *Health Technol Assess.* 2015;19(51):v–xxviii, 1–247.
4. Photocoagulation for diabetic macular edema. Early Treatment Diabetic Retinopathy Study report number 1. Early Treatment Diabetic Retinopathy Study research group. *Arch Ophthalmol.* 1985;103(12):1796–806.
5. Effects of aspirin treatment on diabetic retinopathy. ETDRS report number 8. Early Treatment Diabetic Retinopathy Study Research Group. *Ophthalmology.* 1991;98(5 Suppl):757–65.
6. Royle P, Mistry H, Auguste P, et al. Pan-retinal photocoagulation and other forms of laser treatment and drug therapies for non-proliferative diabetic retinopathy: systematic review and economic evaluation. *Health Technol Assess.* 2015;19(51):v–xxviii, 1–247.
7. Mistry H, Auguste P, Lois N, Waugh N. Diabetic retinopathy and the use of laser photocoagulation: is it cost-effective to treat early? *BMJ Open Ophthalmol.* 2017;2(1):e000021.

31

Does Pars Plana Vitrectomy Improve Visual Outcomes in Patients with Complications of Proliferative Diabetic Retinopathy

Early Treatment Diabetic Retinopathy Study (ETDRS)
Report Number 17[*]

> Pars plana vitrectomy continues to play an important role in the management of complications from proliferative diabetic retinopathy.
> —ETDRS RESEARCH GROUP[1]

Research Questions:
1. How do patient characteristics compare between those needing a pars plana vitrectomy (PPV) and those who do not?
2. Does PPV improve visual outcomes?
3. Does prior scatter laser photocoagulation change the visual outcome in postvitrectomy patients?[1]

Funding: National Eye Institute, National Institutes of Health.

Year Study Began: 1980.

[*] Basic and Clinical Science Course, Section 12. *Retina and Vitreous*. San Francisco: American Academy of Ophthalmology; 2018–2019.

Year Study Published: 1992.

Study Location: 29 centers in the United States.

Who Was Studied: 208 patients (243 eyes) who underwent PPV.

Who Was Excluded: Patients in the ETDRS who did not undergo PPV during the study period.

How Many Patients: 208 (243 eyes).

Study Overview: The ETDRS was a prospective, randomized clinical trial (Figure 31.1).[1,2]

Nearly 4,000 diabetic patients with early proliferative retinopathy, moderate to severe nonproliferative retinopathy, and/or diabetic macular edema in each eye were enrolled. This paper reports the findings in the subgroup of patients in the ETDRS who had PPV and presents baseline previtrectomy characteristics, initial treatment assignments, indications for vitrectomy, and visual outcomes in these patients.

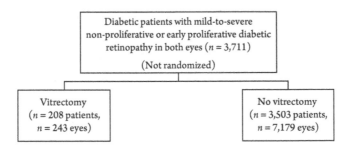

Figure 31.1 Summary of the ETDRS.

Study Intervention: PPV was performed in eyes that had an indication during the study period. These indications included vitreous hemorrhage or retinal detachment with or without vitreous hemorrhage.

Follow-Up: 3 years of follow-up after surgery are available for fewer than 50% of the vitrectomy patients.

Endpoints: Best corrected visual acuity; severe visual loss was defined as a visual acuity of less than 5/200 on 2 consecutive follow-up examinations scheduled at 4-month intervals in patients who underwent PPV.

RESULTS

- Vitrectomy was performed in 208 (5.6%) of the 3,711 patients (243 eyes) enrolled in the ETDRS. Most (52%) had type 1 diabetes; another 35% had a mixed type.
- High-risk proliferative retinopathy was identified before vitrectomy in 91% (221 of 243) of eyes.
  - The indication for vitrectomy in the 243 eyes was vitreous hemorrhage alone in 53.9% of cases and retinal detachment, with or without hemorrhage, in 46.1%.
  - Retinal detachment with or without vitreous hemorrhage was the indication for surgery in 72 (55.0%) of the 131 eyes of type 1 diabetic patients compared with 9 (30.0%) of 30 eyes of type 2 diabetic patients (P =0.024).
- Nearly all eyes undergoing PPV received panretinal photocoagulation treatment (either preoperatively, intraoperatively, or both).
  - Overall, 88% of vitrectomy cases in the ETDRS received prior scatter photocoagulation treatment, including 69.1% (168 of 243) receiving full scatter treatment.
    - Scatter photocoagulation treatment was initiated in 128 (83%) of the 154 eyes assigned to deferral, but only 99 eyes (64%) in the deferral group had received full scatter treatment before the PPV.
    - In the early photocoagulation treatment group, 69 of 89 eyes (78%) received full scatter prior to vitrectomy.
  - The 5-year vitrectomy rates were 2.1% in eyes assigned to early full scatter photocoagulation as the initial treatment, 2.5% in eyes assigned to early mild scatter photocoagulation, and 4.0% in eyes assigned to deferral.
  - The postvitrectomy visual acuity results comparing eyes that received either less than full scatter (<1,200 burns) or no photocoagulation with eyes that received full scatter panretinal photocoagulation before vitrectomy showed no statistically significant difference.
  - Comparison of postvitrectomy visual acuity results between eyes assigned to deferral of photocoagulation and eyes assigned to early photocoagulation also showed no statistically significant difference.
- Before vitrectomy, visual acuity was 5/200 or worse in 66.7% of eyes and better than 20/100 in 6.2%.
  - One year after vitrectomy, the visual acuity was 20/100 or better in 47.6% of eyes, including 24.0% with visual acuity of 20/40 or better.

- These levels of visual acuity remained essentially constant during the 3 years of follow-up.
- The percentage of eyes with less than 5/200 visual acuity after vitrectomy were 20.2% (year 1), 24.7% (year 2), and 27.7% (year 3).
- Neovascular glaucoma occurred in 1.5% of eyes in the nonvitrectomy group and 12.8% of eyes that had a vitrectomy.

Criticisms and Limitations: ETDRS patients undergoing vitrectomy were generally white (76%), and were more likely to have type 1 diabetes (52%) and poorer control, thus the outcomes may not translate exactly to other demographic/clinical groups.

Complete information concerning the details of the macular status and intraoperative complications was not available as one third of the operative notes were either missing or incomplete.

Other Relevant Studies and Information:

- Aspirin use did not lead to a higher rate of vitrectomy, either in the overall group or in the subgroup of patients with vitreous hemorrhage.
  - The 5-year vitrectomy rates (vitrectomy in either eye) for patients assigned to aspirin (5.4%) versus those assigned to placebo (5.2%) showed no statistically significant difference ($P = 0.91$).
- Technological advances in PPV since the ETDRS include microincisional vitrectomy technology, wide angle microscope viewing systems, and adjunctive pharmacologic agents.[3,4]
- In vitreous hemorrhage where PRP cannot be performed, use of anti–vascular endothelial growth factor medications can treat underlying PDR and delay or reduce need for vitrectomy.[5]

Summary and Implications: Pars plana vitrectomy continues to play an important role in the management of complications from proliferative diabetic retinopathy. Adverse events from PDR can occur despite early photocoagulation treatment. Provided there were good anatomic and visual acuity results 6 months after vitrectomy, the visual acuity results tended to remain stable for up to 10 years of follow-up. There are no ocular contraindications to aspirin when required for cardiovascular disease or other medical problems.

CLINICAL CASE: COUNSELING A PATIENT WITH PROLIFERATIVE DIABETIC RETINOPATHY

Case History

A 52-year-old Caucasian man presents to your clinic for a follow-up visit. He has a past medical history of type 1 diabetes that has been poorly controlled and high blood pressure. In addition to medications he takes for these conditions, he also takes a daily aspirin as prescribed by his primary physician. He has previously received full scatter laser photocoagulation treatment (as defined by ETDRS) for severe nonproliferative diabetic retinopathy. Today you are seeing him at a 1-month follow-up for a nonresolving vitreous hemorrhage in the right eye. His vision in that eye is 20/400. You recommend he undergo a PPV. The patient asks about his "chances" if he proceeds with surgery. According to the ETDRS Report 17, which of the following statements is true?

A. The ETDRS found a statistically significant chance of better visual acuity after the PPV in patients who had previously undergone full scatter laser photocoagulation compared with patients who had no photocoagulation before PPV.
B. The ETDRS found that patients who were not taking aspirin as prescribed by their primary physicians had a statistically significant decrease in their need for PPV.
C. The ETDRS found that a smaller percentage of patients that underwent PPV developed neovascular glaucoma compared with patients who did not have a vitrectomy.
D. The ETDRS found that 1 year after vitrectomy, visual acuity was 20/100 or better in nearly half of treated eyes.

Suggested Answer

Option D.

References

1. Flynn HW Jr, Chew EY, Simons BD, Barton FB, Remaley NA, Ferris FL 3rd. Pars plana vitrectomy in the Early Treatment Diabetic Retinopathy Study. ETDRS report number 17. The Early Treatment Diabetic Retinopathy Study Research Group. *Ophthalmology*. 1992;99(9):1351–57.
2. Early Treatment Diabetic Retinopathy Study design and baseline patient characteristics. ETDRS report number 7. *Ophthalmology*. 1991;98(5 Suppl):741–56.

3. Cruz-Iñigo YJ, Acabá LA, Berrocal MH. Surgical management of retinal diseases: proliferative diabetic retinopathy and traction retinal detachment. *Dev Ophthalmol.* 2014;54:196–203.
4. Berrocal MH, Acaba LA, Acaba A. Surgery for diabetic eye complications. *Curr Diab Rep.* 2016;16(10):99.
5. Zhao Y, Singh RP. The role of anti-vascular endothelial growth factor (anti-VEGF) in the management of proliferative diabetic retinopathy. *Drugs Context.* 2018;7:212532.

32

Intensive Diabetes Management to Reduce the Risk of Retinopathy Developing or Progressing*

The Diabetes Control and Complications Trial (DCCT)

> Although intensive therapy does not prevent retinopathy completely, it has a beneficial effect that begins after 3 years of therapy on all levels of retinopathy studied in the DCCT.
>
> —DCCT RESEARCH GROUP[1]

Research Questions:

1. Does intensive therapy completely prevent the development of retinopathy?
2. Are some states of retinopathy too advanced to benefit from intensive therapy?
3. Are the retinopathy endpoints in the DCCT clinically important?
4. What other factors influence the effectiveness of therapy?[1]

Funding: Division of Diabetes, Endocrinology, and Metabolic Diseases, National Institute of Diabetes and Digestive and Kidney Diseases; National

---

* Basic and Clinical Science Course, Section 12. *Retina and Vitreous.* San Francisco: American Academy of Ophthalmology; 2018–2019: 95–98.

Eye Institute; National Heart, Lung and Blood Institute; National Center for Research Resources (all National Institutes of Health).

Year Study Began: 1983.

Year Study Published: 1995.

Study Location: 29 centers in the United States and Canada.

Who Was Studied: For the primary prevention cohort: patients between the ages of 13 and 39 years with insulin-dependent diabetes mellitus (IDDM) of 1 to 5 years' duration and no retinopathy or microalbuminuria at baseline. For the secondary intervention cohort: patients between the ages of 13 and 39 years with IDDM of 1 to 15 years' duration, minimal to moderate nonproliferative retinopathy (at least one microaneurysm in either eye), and an albuminuria level <200 mg/24 hours.

Who Was Excluded: Persons with hypertension, hypercholesterolemia, severe diabetic complications, or medical conditions such as cardiovascular disease.

How Many Patients: 1,441.

Study Overview: The Diabetes Control and Complications Trial was a randomized clinical trial (Figure 32.1).[1-3]

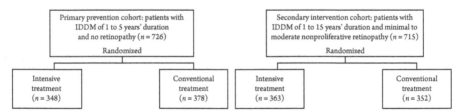

Figure 32.1 Summary of the DCCT.

Study Intervention: Patients in the primary prevention cohort were randomly allocated to receive conventional or intensive treatment; patients in the secondary intervention cohort were randomly assigned similarly. Intensive therapy, aimed at achieving glycemic levels as close to the normal range as possible, included three or more daily insulin injections or a continuous subcutaneous insulin infusion, guided by four or more glucose tests daily, with the goal of achieving and maintaining glycemic control as near normal as possible while avoiding severe hypoglycemia. The conventional therapy group was given up to two injections daily of any mixture of short-acting, intermediate, or long-acting insulin with no predefined targets for glucose control being identified; the goal was the absence of symptoms of hyperglycemia or hypoglycemia, absence of ketonuria, and maintenance of normal growth and development.

Follow-Up: Patients in the primary prevention cohort were followed for an average of 6.0 years, and those in the secondary intervention cohort were followed for 7.0 years.

Endpoints: The primary prevention cohort's principal outcome was the sustained development of retinopathy, defined as at least 1 microaneurysm in two consecutive 6-month sets of photographs. The secondary intervention cohort's principal outcome was a three or more step progression in retinopathy as judged by the Early Treatment Diabetic Retinopathy Study (ETDRS) protocol for grading retinopathy. Renal and cardiovascular outcomes were also assessed.

RESULTS

Primary Prevention Cohort
- Both treatment groups had a steady rise in cumulative incidence of sustained microaneurysms; the intensively treated group had a relatively lower rate beginning after 3 years of follow-up.
  - The cumulative incidence of sustained microaneurysms was nearly 70% in the intensive treatment group, versus 90% in the conventional therapy group.
  - Sustained microaneurysms developed at an average rate of 14.9 cases per 100 patient-years in patients who had undergone intensive treatment versus 19.8 per 100 patient-years among patients who received conventional treatment (average risk reduction over 9 years = 27%; $P = .002$).
  - Using a more conservative definition of retinopathy requiring a three or more step progression over 9 years, the risk reduction increased to 76%.

Secondary Intervention Cohort
- The 9-year cumulative incidence of three or more step progression was 56% in patients who received intensive treatment versus 78% in those who were treated conventionally, a risk reduction of 34% with intensive treatment.

- Over 9 years, the cumulative incidence of sustained 3 or more step progression as defined by the final ETDRS scale was 17% with intensive treatment compared to 49% with conventional treatment, an average risk reduction of 65%.
- The 9-year cumulative incidence of severe nonproliferative retinopathy was 9.2% for patients who received intensive treatment and 26% for those who received conventional treatment, an average risk reduction of 47%.
- The 9-year incidence rates for new vessels on the disc and/or new vessels elsewhere were 24% and 8%, respectively, for patients who received conventional and intensive treatment, a risk reduction of 48% with intensive therapy.
- For macular edema, the cumulative incidence over 9 years was estimated to be 27% among patients who received intensive treatment, versus 44% among those who received conventional treatment, a risk reduction of 29% $(P = 0.025)$.
  - The cumulative incidence of clinically significant macular edema was estimated to be 15% and 27% in the two groups, respectively, a risk reduction of 23%, the latter not statistically significant.
- Overall, intensive therapy slowed progression of retinopathy by 54%.
- Over 9 years, an estimated 7.9 of subjects who received intensive treatment would require at least one episode of laser treatment, versus approximately 30% of those who received conventional treatment, a risk reduction of 59% $(P = 0.001)$.
- Although the mortality did not differ significantly between treatment groups, patients in the intensive treatment group were approximately 3 times more likely to experience an episode of hypoglycemia than those in the conventional treatment group.

Criticisms and Limitations: Patients with non-insulin-dependent diabetes mellitus (NIDDM) were not studied during this trial, making it difficult to extrapolate the results of this trial to patients with NIDDM.

Patients with severe nonproliferative or proliferative diabetic retinopathy were also excluded from the study; they may be at higher risk for progression of their retinopathy after initiation of intensive therapy.

The intensive therapy regimen carried out during this trial required extensive use of medical resources, including the services of physicians, nurses, dietitians, and behavioral specialists. Therefore, alternative strategies to adapt this intensive regimen for the general population would be necessary.

Other Relevant Studies and Information:

- As described in an earlier DCCT report, there is a transient worsening of diabetic retinopathy with intensive therapy, which delays the appearance of a benefit during the first 2 years of treatment. This was mostly seen in patients in the secondary intervention cohort, and these findings often disappeared by 18 months.[4]
- At the conclusion of the DCCT, the cohort of >1,400 patients was followed in a longitudinal observation study known as the Epidemiology of Diabetes Interventions and Complications (EDIC) study, in which the patients in the conventional treatment group were converted to intensive treatment and followed for many years.[5]
- Mean HbA1c levels during the DCCT trial were 9.1% and 7.2% for conventional and intensive treatment, respectively. During the EDIC study, the difference in HbA1c levels between groups disappeared over time as all patients adopted the intensive regimen; however, over the first four years of EDIC, further widening of the differences in outcomes between intensive and conventional treatment groups was observed, indicating a "metabolic memory" which was seen in all microvascular complications.

Summary and Implications: Although intensive therapy in patients with IDDM does not prevent retinopathy completely, it reduces the risk of retinopathy developing or progressing, especially when started early in the course of IDDM. Intensive therapy has a beneficial effect that begins after 3 years on all levels of retinopathy. Even in patients with nonproliferative retinopathy of moderate severity, retinopathy is more likely to regress or remain unchanged over time with intensive therapy. All eye care specialists should educate their diabetic patients about the importance of achieving glycemic levels as close to the normal range as possible, to reduce the risk of visual loss and the need for laser treatment.

CLINICAL CASE: A YOUNG MAN WITH EARLY DIABETIC RETINOPATHY

Case History
A 22-year-old white man with a past medical history of type 1 diabetes of 5 years' duration presents to your clinic for his first eye exam in 3 years. He is

prescribed long-acting insulin nightly and short-acting insulin with meals. He states that he forgets to take his insulin a few times a week, but he has not experienced any symptoms of hypoglycemia or hyperglycemia recently. His last HbA1c was 9.1% five months ago. He has occasional floaters in both eyes, but denies any new showers of floaters, flashes of light, or curtains of vision loss. He has no other visual complaints, but states that his feet "fall asleep" regularly. He also takes loratadine over-the-counter for seasonal allergies. He drinks alcohol 3–4 times a week "socially" and denies any tobacco or illicit drug use.

On examination, visual acuity is 20/30 in the right eye and 20/25 in the left eye. His pupils are equal, round, and reactive to light and accommodation. Extraocular movements appear normal and confrontational visual fields are full in both eyes. Intraocular pressures are 16 mm Hg in the right eye and 12 mm Hg in the left eye. External, lid, and anterior segment examination of both eyes is unremarkable. Dilated fundus exam reveals microaneurysms and cotton-wool spots in both eyes. The right eye also has two small hard exudates. There are no obvious retinal hemorrhages or intraretinal microvascular abnormalities. Both optic nerves have a cup-to-disc ratio of 0.25, and the retinal vessels appear normal in both eyes. The patient is informed of these findings and asks what he can do to stop the progression of diabetic retinopathy. What is the clinician's best response to the patient's inquiry?

A. Continue the current treatment regimen, as the patient is not experiencing any adverse symptoms.
B. Regardless of treatment, his diabetic retinopathy will undoubtedly progress.
C. Referral to the patient's primary care physician to answer questions regarding diabetic complications.
D. Encourage intensive diabetic treatment with strict glycemic control.

Suggested Answer

The history and examination findings in this patient are suggestive of diabetic retinopathy. Based on the results of the DCCT, the patient should undergo intensive diabetic treatment with strict glycemic control (option D) to slow the progression of diabetic retinopathy.

References

1. Progression of retinopathy with intensive versus conventional treatment in the Diabetes Control and Complications Trial. Diabetes Control and Complications Trial Research Group. *Ophthalmology*. 1995;102(4):647–61.

2. The DCCT Research Group. The Diabetes Control and Complications Trial (DCCT). Design and methodologic considerations for the feasibility phase. *Diabetes.* 1986;35(5):530–45.
3. The DCCT Research Group. The Diabetes Control and Complications Trial DCCT: update. *Diabetes Care.* 1990;13(4):427–33.
4. Diabetes Control and Complications Trial Research Group, Nathan DM, Genuth S, Lachin J, et al. The effect of intensive treatment of diabetes on the development and progression of long-term complications in insulin-dependent diabetes mellitus. *N Engl J Med.* 1993;329(14):977–86.
5. Nathan DM. The Diabetes Control and Complications Trial/Epidemiology of Diabetes Interventions and Complications Study at 30 years: overview. The DCCT/EDIC Research Group. *Diabetes Care.* 2014;37(1):9–16.

33

Progression of Retinopathy and Vision Loss Related to Tight Blood Pressure Control in Type 2 Diabetes Mellitus*

UK Prospective Diabetes Study (UKPDS) Hypertension in Diabetes Study

High blood pressure is detrimental to each aspect of diabetic retinopathy; a tight blood pressure control policy reduces the risk of clinical complications from diabetic eye disease.

—UKPDS Group[1]

Research Question: What is the relationship between tight blood pressure (BP) control and the different aspects of diabetic retinopathy in patients with type 2 diabetes mellitus?[1]

Funding: United Kingdom (UK) Medical Research Council, London, England; British Diabetic Association; UK Department of Health, London; National Eye Institute, National Institute of Digestive, Diabetes, and Kidney Disease in the National Institutes of Health, Bethesda, MD; British Heart Foundation,

---

* Basic and Clinical Science Course, Section 12. *Retina and Vitreous*. San Francisco: American Academy of Ophthalmology; 2018–2019: 96–98.

London; Novo-Nordisk A/S, Copenhagen, Denmark; Bayer (Schweiz) AG, Zurich, Switzerland; Bristol-Myers Squibb, New York, NY; Hoechst AG, Kehl, Germany; Eli Lilly & Co, Indianapolis, IN; Lipha and Farmitalia Carlo Erba, Milan, Italy.

Year Study Began: The UKPDS began in 1977; the Hypertension in Diabetes Study was started in 1987.

Year Study Published: 2004.

Study Location: 19 hospital-based clinics in England, Scotland, and Northern Ireland.

Who Was Studied: Newly diagnosed patients, aged 25–65 years inclusive, with type 2 (non-insulin-dependent) diabetes mellitus and hypertension. Diabetes was defined as persistent hyperglycemia (fasting plasma glucose level, 110–270 mg/dL [6.1–15.0 mmol/L]) on treatment with diet alone for 3 months. Hypertension was defined as a systolic blood pressure (SBP) 160 mm Hg or higher and/or a diastolic (DBP) 90 mm Hg or higher (if not receiving treatment for hypertension) or an SBP 150 mm Hg or higher and/or a DBP 85 mm Hg or higher (if already receiving treatment for hypertension).

Who Was Excluded: Patients with a clinical requirement for strict BP control (previous stroke, accelerated hypertension, cardiac failure, or renal failure) or beta-blockade (myocardial infarction in the previous year or current angina); severe vascular disease; a severe concurrent illness or contraindications to beta-blockers. Those with malignant hypertension and those with preexisting retinopathy needing laser treatment were also excluded.

How Many Patients: 1,148.

Study Overview: The UKPDS was a prospective, randomized, intervention trial in patients with type 2 (non-insulin-dependent) diabetes mellitus to determine whether improved blood glucose control prevented complications and reduced the associated morbidity and mortality.[1,2] The Hypertension in Diabetes Study, reported in this paper, was included in a factorial design to assess whether improved BP control would be advantageous (Figure 33.1).

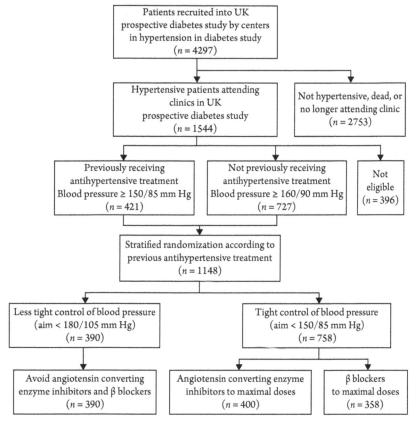

Figure 33.1 Summary of the UKPDS Hypertension in Diabetes study.

Study Intervention: In the main randomization, those who were asymptomatic and had fasting plasma glucose under 15 mmol/l were allocated either to diet policy, or to active policy with either insulin or sulphonylurea aiming to reduce the fasting plasma glucose to under 6 mmol/l. In the Hypertension in Diabetes Study, patients with hypertension were randomly allocated between a less tight BP control policy, aiming for an SBP less than 180 mm Hg and a DBP less than 105 mm Hg, and a tight BP control policy, with a random allocation to either an angiotensin-converting enzyme (ACE) inhibitor or a beta-blocker, aiming for an SBP less than 150 and a DBP less than 85 mm Hg.

Follow-Up: Median follow-up was 8.4 years.

Endpoints: Deterioration of retinopathy (≥2-step change on a modified Early Treatment Diabetic Retinopathy Study [ETDRS] final scale), together with endpoints (photocoagulation, vitreous hemorrhage, and cataract extraction) and analysis of specific lesions (microaneurysms, hard exudates, and cotton-wool spots). Blindness was monitored as an endpoint with the criterion of Snellen chart assessment at 6/60 or worse. (The reasons for visual loss were not prospectively collected in the UKPDS data set and were assessed from ophthalmic notes, where available, retrospectively.)

RESULTS

- The mean cohort BP during the study over 9 years follow-up was 144/ 82 mm Hg for the tight BP control group and 154/87 mm Hg for the less tight BP group (each $P < .001$).
- The mean glycosylated hemoglobin level A1c over years 1 through 4 was 7.2% in both groups and over years 5 through 8 was 8.3% and 8.2% in the tight and less tight BP groups, respectively.
- At 4.5 years, there was a highly significant difference in microaneurysm count, with 23.3% in the tight BP control group and 33.5%in the less tight BP control group having 5 or more microaneurysms (relative risk [RR], 0.70; $P = .003$).
  - The effect continued to 7.5 years (RR, 0.66; $P < .001$).
  - The difference at 7.5 years was seen in both the primary prevention cohort (RR, 0.64; $P = .053$) and the secondary prevention cohort (RR, 0.73; $P = .046$).
- Hard exudates increased over time in both groups, from a prevalence of 11.2% to 18.3% at 7.5 years after randomization, with fewer lesions found in the tight BP control group (RR, 0.53; $P < .001$).
- Cotton-wool spots increased over time in both groups but less so in the tight BP control group, which had fewer cotton-wool spots at 7.5 years (RR, 0.53; $P < .001$).
- A 2-step or more deterioration on the ETDRS scale was significantly different at 4.5 years, with fewer people in the tight BP control group progressing 2 steps or more (RR, 0.75; $P = .02$).
  - This was more marked at 7.5 years (RR, 0.66; $P < .001$).
  - The difference at 7.5 years was seen in both the primary prevention and the secondary prevention cohorts.
- Patients allocated to tight BP control were less likely to undergo photocoagulation (RR, 0.65; $P = .03$).
  - This difference was driven by a difference in photocoagulation due to maculopathy (RR, 0.58; $P = .02$).

- Five patients had a vitreous hemorrhage: 3 in the tight BP control group and 2 in the less tight BP control group (too few events to analyze statistically).
- The tight BP control group compared with the less tight BP control group had a 47% lower risk of a deterioration in visual acuity by 3 or more lines ($P = .004$) on a Snellen visual acuity chart.
- The cumulative incidence of the end point of blindness (Snellen visual acuity, ≥6/60) in 1 eye was 18/758 (2.4%) for the tight BP control group compared with 12/390 (3.1%) for less tight BP control group. These equate to absolute risks of 3.1 to 4.1 per 1,000 patient-years, respectively ($P = .046$; RR, 0.76).
- There was no detectable difference in outcomes (microaneurysms, hard exudates, cotton-wool spots, frequency of photocoagulation, blindness) between the 2 randomized therapies of ACE inhibition and beta-blockade.

Criticisms and Limitations: There were few nonwhites in the study, and the eldest subjects were 65 years of age at recruitment, so generalization of the results to other racial/ethnic groups and older age groups may be limited.

The patients studied had a relatively short duration of type 2 diabetes and moderate to severe hypertension. The efficacy of lowering BP in persons with mild hypertension, who are normotensive, who have longer duration or more severe retinopathy, or who have type 1 diabetes may be different. Furthermore, since the UKPDS, newer/different classes of antihypertensive drug have been developed with greater efficacy than those used in the UKPDS.[3]

Patients were reviewed 3-monthly, rather than 6–12 monthly as in routine clinical practice, which may have improved compliance and optimized the results.

Other Relevant Studies and Information:

- The Diabetes Control and Complications Trial (DCCT) showed that intensive treatment with the goal of maintaining blood glucose concentrations close to the normal range effectively delayed the onset and slowed the progression of diabetic retinopathy in patients with IDDM, although it did not prevent retinopathy completely.[4,5]
- Earlier reports from the UKPDS showed that in patients with type 2 diabetes the risk of diabetic complications was strongly associated with raised blood pressure, with the lowest risk being in those with systolic blood pressure less than 120 mm Hg, and that tight blood pressure control in patients with hypertension and type 2 diabetes achieved a

clinically important reduction in the risk of deaths related to diabetes, complications related to diabetes, progression of diabetic retinopathy, and deterioration in visual acuity.[6,7]

- After 9 years the group assigned to tight BP control had 37% reduction in risk of microvascular end points (11% to 56%) ($P = .0092$), predominantly owing to a reduced risk of retinal photocoagulation for sight-threatening retinopathy, diabetic macular edema, and proliferative retinopathy.[6]

- The Appropriate Blood Pressure Control in Diabetes (ABCD) Trial, a prospective randomized blinded clinical trial to compare the effects of intensive versus moderate blood pressure control on the incidence and progression of type 2 diabetic complications in persons with type 2 diabetes and hypertension (defined as DBP ≥ 90 mm Hg), found that over a 5-year follow-up period, there was no difference between the intensive and moderate groups with regard to the progression of diabetic retinopathy; in addition, the use of nisoldipine versus enalapril had no differential effect on diabetic retinopathy.[8]

  - However, in normotensive (BP <140/90 mm Hg) type 2 diabetic patients, the intensive BP control group (mean BP approximately 128/75 mm Hg) demonstrated less progression of diabetic retinopathy (34% vs. 46%; $P = .02$) than the moderate therapy group, with no difference whether enalapril or nisoldipine was used as the initial antihypertensive agent.[9]

  - These data from the UKPDS and ABCD groups suggest that in persons with type 2 diabetes there is no threshold effect below which further reduction of blood pressure lacks efficacy.

- The EURODIAB Controlled Trial of Lisinopril in Insulin Dependent Diabetes Mellitus, a randomized double-blind placebo-controlled trial of the efficacy of blood pressure lowering with lisinopril on retinopathy in persons with type 1 diabetes, showed a statistically significant 50% reduction in the progression of retinopathy in those taking lisinopril during a 2-year period. This finding was independent of glycemic control. The finding was not significant after controlling for study center ($P = .06$).[10]

Summary and Implications: The UKPDS Hypertension in Diabetes Study findings clearly demonstrate the importance of lowering blood pressure to reduce the progression of retinopathy, incidence of macular edema, and loss of vision in persons with relatively short duration of type 2 diabetes and moderate to severe hypertension. Treatment begun early in the course of type 2 diabetes is likely to have a long-term effect of reducing visual loss secondary to diabetic macular edema in persons with type 2 diabetes. Ophthalmologists should tell their diabetic patients about the benefits of blood pressure control in reducing loss of vision from diabetic retinopathy and emphasize the need for routine monitoring of blood pressure (including measurements at each eye examination).

CLINICAL CASE: AN ELDERLY WOMAN WITH DIABETES, HYPERTENSION, AND DIABETIC RETINOPATHY

Case History
A 66-year-old African American woman with a past medical history of type 2 diabetes and hypertension presents to your clinic complaining of blurring of vision in the right eye for the past 3 days. She is a known case of moderate diabetic retinopathy in both eyes but was lost to follow-up. On exam today she has severe nonproliferative diabetic retinopathy with macular edema in the right eye and severe nonproliferative diabetic retinopathy without macular edema in the left eye. According to the UKPDS trial, tight control of BP will:

A. Increase her chances of receiving photocoagulation for maculopathy.
B. Decrease her chances of receiving photocoagulation for maculopathy.
C. Have no impact on her chances of receiving photocoagulation.
D. Reduce the development of microaneurysms and hard exudates but will not prevent visual deterioration.

Suggested Answer
The correct answer is B. According to the UKPDS, patients allocated to tight BP control were less likely to undergo photocoagulation, largely due to the benefits of photocoagulation for maculopathy.

References

1. Matthews DR, Stratton IM, Aldington SJ, Holman RR, Kohner EM; UK Prospective Diabetes Study Group. Risks of progression of retinopathy and vision loss related to tight blood pressure control in type 2 diabetes mellitus: UKPDS 69. *Arch Ophthalmol.* 2004;122(11):1631–40.

2. UK Prospective Diabetes Study (UKPDS). VIII. Study design, progress and performance. *Diabetologia*. 1991;34(12):877–90.
3. Klein R. Is intensive management of blood pressure to prevent visual loss in persons with type 2 diabetes indicated? *Arch Ophthalmol*. 2004;122(11):1707–9.
4. Diabetes Control and Complications Trial Research Group, Nathan DM, Genuth S, Lachin J, et al. The effect of intensive treatment of diabetes on the development and progression of long-term complications in insulin-dependent diabetes mellitus. *N Engl J Med*. 1993;329(14):977–86.
5. Progression of retinopathy with intensive versus conventional treatment in the Diabetes Control and Complications Trial. Diabetes Control and Complications Trial Research Group. *Ophthalmology*. 1995;102(4):647–61.
6. Tight blood pressure control and risk of macrovascular and microvascular complications in type 2 diabetes: UKPDS 38. UK Prospective Diabetes Study Group. *BMJ*. 1998;317(7160):703–13.
7. Adler AI, Stratton IM, Neil HA, et al. Association of systolic blood pressure with macrovascular and microvascular complications of type 2 diabetes (UKPDS 36): prospective observational study. *BMJ*. 2000;321(7258):412–9.
8. Estacio RO, Jeffers BW, Gifford N, Schrier RW. Effect of blood pressure control on diabetic microvascular complications in patients with hypertension and type 2 diabetes. *Diabetes Care*. 2000;23(Suppl 2):B54–B64.
9. Schrier RW, Estacio RO, Esler A, Mehler P. Effects of aggressive blood pressure control in normotensive type 2 diabetic patients on albuminuria, retinopathy, and strokes. *Kidney Int*. 2002;61(3):1086–97.
10. Chaturvedi N, Sjolie AK, Stephenson JM, et al. Effect of lisinopril on progression of retinopathy in normotensive people with type 1 diabetes: the EUCLID Study Group. EURODIAB Controlled Trial of Lisinopril in Insulin-Dependent Diabetes Mellitus. *Lancet*. 1998;351(9095):28–31.

34

Immediate Vitrectomy and Intravenous Antibiotics for the Treatment of Postoperative Bacterial Endophthalmitis[*]

Endophthalmitis Vitrectomy Study (EVS)

Omission of systemic antibiotic treatment can reduce toxic effects, costs, and length of hospital stay. Routine immediate pars plana vitrectomy is not necessary in patient with better than light perception vision at presentation but is of substantial benefit for those who have light perception-only vision.

—EVS GROUP[1]

Research Question: What are the roles of immediate pars plana vitrectomy (VIT) and systemic antibiotic treatment in the management of postoperative endophthalmitis?[1]

Funding: National Eye Institute, National Institutes of Health.

Year Study Began: 1990.

Year Study Published: 1995.

---

[*] Basic and Clinical Science Course, Section 12. *Retina and Vitreous.* San Francisco: American Academy of Ophthalmology; 2018–2019: 389–390.

Study Location: 24 practices in the United States.

Who Was Studied: Patients, 18 years of age and older, with clinical signs and symptoms of bacterial endophthalmitis within 6 weeks of cataract surgery or secondary lens implantation. Eligibility required visual acuity of between 20/50 and light perception (LP), plus clear enough cornea and anterior chamber for visualization of some portion of the iris, a clear enough cornea in order to perform VIT, and the presence of hypopyon or clouding of the anterior chamber or vitreous that obscured the view of second-order retinal arterioles.

Who Was Excluded: Patient were excluded if they had previous eye disease limiting visual acuity to ≤20/100 before cataract development, prior intraocular surgery aside from cataract or secondary lens implantation, previous penetrating ocular injury, past intravitreal antibiotic injection or VIT, retinal or choroidal detachment that was moderate in height as judged by ultrasound or indirect ophthalmoscopy, or suspicion for fungal endophthalmitis.

How Many Patients: 420.

Study Overview: The EVS was a randomized, controlled clinical trial (Figure 34.1).[1]

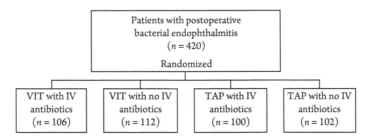

Figure 34.1 Summary of EVS.

Study Intervention: Using a 2 × 2 factorial design, patients were split into the following four groups: vitreous tap/biopsy (TAP) with IV antibiotics, pars plana vitrectomy (VIT) with IV antibiotics, TAP without IV antibiotics, and VIT without IV antibiotics. The TAP group underwent trans–pars plana vitreous needle aspiration or vitreous biopsy through a single sclerotomy using a VIT instrument. All patients received an anterior chamber biopsy (0.1 mL) with 25 or 27 g needle. Two antibiotics were given intravenously: first, ceftazidime, 2 g every 8 hours (1.5 g for patients weighing less than 50 kg) or ciprofloxacin 750 mg by mouth twice daily in patients with penicillin allergies; the second drug was amikacin in a 7.5 mg/kg initial dosing, followed by 6 mg/kg every twice a day with doses adjusted based off blood concentration.

After either VIT or TAP, all patients received intravitreal injections of amikacin 0.4 mg in 0.1 mL solution and vancomycin hydrochloride (1.0 mg in 0.1 mL). They also received subconjunctival injections ceftazidime (100 mg in 0.5 mL), vancomycin hydrochloride (25 mg in 0.5 mL), and dexamethasone sodium phosphate (6 mg in 0.25 mL). If penicillin allergy was present, amikacin (25 mg in 0.5 mL) was given subconjunctivally instead of ceftazidime. Topical vancomycin and amikacin were given every 4 hours or as often as every hour if wound leak or wound infection was present. Topical 1% atropine or 0.25% scopolamine and topical 1% prednisolone acetate were given after surgery. Oral prednisone 30 mg twice daily for 5 to 10 days was also given to all patients.

Patients in the TAP group were allowed to have VIT with reinjection of intravitreal antibiotics if the eye was doing poorly after 36 to 60 hours. Patients in the VIT group were also allowed repeated VIT with reinjection of intravitreal antibiotics.

Follow-Up: 9 months.

Endpoints: The primary outcome measures were visual acuity and clarity of the ocular media.

RESULTS

- The median time from the cataract extraction or secondary lens implantation until presentation to a study center was 6 days; presentation within 2 to 6 weeks occurred in 22%.
- At baseline, 86% had visual acuity of less than 5/200; visual acuity was LP only in 26% of patients.
  - Media clarity at the initial visit was poor: in almost 80% of patients, no retinal vessel of any type could be seen with indirect ophthalmoscopy. A red reflex was absent in 67% of patients.
- Overall, more than half of the patients achieved 20/40 vision, and three-quarters achieved 20/100 or better visual outcome, regardless of treatment. Only 11% of patients had final visual acuity worse than 5/200.
- There was no difference in final visual acuity or media clarity with or without the use of systemic antibiotics.
- In patients whose initial visual acuity was hand motions or better, there was no difference in visual outcome whether or not an immediate VIT was performed.
  - Patients who initially had HM vision or better had the same chance of attaining >20/40 visual acuity (66% vs. 62%) and >20/100 acuity

(86% vs. 84%) and a comparable risk for visual acuity loss <5/200 (5% vs. 3%).

- The benefit of VIT was limited to patients who had initial vision of LP-only or worse. In this group, those who underwent VIT had 3 times higher chance of attaining ≥20/40 final visual acuity (33% vs. 11%), nearly double the chance of attaining ≥20/100 final visual acuity (56% vs. 30%), and less than half the risk for severe visual acuity loss of <5/200 (20% vs. 47%), compared to TAP.
- At 3 months, clearing of the ocular media occurred in 86% of those having VIT, compared to 75% in those having TAP ($P = .004$); at the 9-month follow-up, the difference was less obvious: VIT—90%, TAP—83%.
  - In the IV antibiotic treatment group, there was no difference in clarity of ocular media.

Criticisms and Limitations: The EVS study evaluated only the use of systemic amikacin and ceftazidime, and could not address the benefits of treatment with other or additional antimicrobial agents.

Subjects with significant opacification of the anterior chamber or without light perception—that is, eyes with more severe infection or involving more virulent organisms—were excluded from the EVS, which might have shifted the EVS outcomes to more favorable results.[2]

The conclusions of the EVS study do not apply to infections that are associated with filtering blebs, are delayed after cataract surgery, follow trauma, or are metastatic from an endogenous source, which may produce a different and more virulent spectrum of organisms. The use of systemic antibiotics remains the standard of care for posttraumatic endophthalmitis and is also necessary for most cases of endogenous endophthalmitis.[3]

Other Relevant Studies and Information:

- Fifty-eight of 420 study patients had diabetes. Diabetic patients had slightly worse vision and ocular media at the baseline assessment. Only 39% of diabetic patients compared with 55% of nondiabetic patients achieved 20/40 final vision. Both diabetic and nondiabetic patients with initial LP-only vision had better visual results with immediate vitrectomy. For those with better than LP baseline vision, patients with diabetes achieved visual acuity of 20/40 more often with vitrectomy (57%) than with TAP (40%), but this difference was not statistically significant. Patients without diabetes did equally well with VIT or TAP.[4]

There were, however, not enough patients with diabetes to determine the optimal management for this group.

Summary and Implications: For endophthalmitis after cataract or secondary IOL surgery, pars plana VIT is recommended in patients with LP vision or worse. TAP is recommended in patients with vision better than LP. Most patients do not require treatment with IV antibiotics.

CLINICAL CASE: A MIDDLE-AGED MAN WITH ENDOPHTHALMITIS AFTER CATARACT SURGERY

Case History

A 61-year-old man presents to the clinic with complaints of severe throbbing eye pain and a sudden drop in vision 6 days after cataract extraction and IOL implantation in the left eye. Baseline exam reveals light perception vision and intraocular pressure of 25 mm Hg. Slit-lamp exam shows a 1.5-mm hypopyon, hazy iris details, and mild corneal edema. Based on the results of the EVS, what would be the recommended intervention for this patient?

A. AC tap with injection of intravitreal antibiotics.
B. Surgical removal of the IOL.
C. IV antibiotics.
D. Pars plana VIT with injections.

Suggested Answer

The above patient likely has postop endophthalmitis, given the recent time frame (6 days) after cataract surgery. Based on the results of the EVS, this patient would benefit from a pars plana VIT with intravitreal antibiotics (option D). IV antibiotics do not play a role in postop endophthalmitis after cataract surgery.

References

1. Results of the Endophthalmitis Vitrectomy Study. A randomized trial of immediate vitrectomy and of intravenous antibiotics for the treatment of postoperative bacterial endophthalmitis. Endophthalmitis Vitrectomy Study Group. *Arch Ophthalmol.* 1995;113(12):1479–96.

2. Flynn HW Jr, Scott IU. Legacy of the endophthalmitis vitrectomy study. *Arch Ophthalmol.* 2008;126(4):559–61.
3. Sternberg P Jr, Martin DF. Management of endophthalmitis in the post-endophthalmitis vitrectomy study era. *Arch Ophthalmol.* 2001;119(5):754–5.
4. Doft BH, Wisniewski SR, Kelsey SF, Fitzgerald SG; Endophthalmitis Vitrectomy Study Group. Diabetes and postoperative endophthalmitis in the endophthalmitis vitrectomy study. *Arch Ophthalmol.* 2001;119(5):650–6.

35

Prevalence of Age-Related Maculopathy*

The Beaver Dam Eye Study

Women over 75 years old are more likely to have exudative age-related macular degeneration (ARMD) when compared with men of their same age group.

—KLEIN ET AL[1]

Research Question: What is the prevalence of macular degeneration and its characteristics in the United States?[1]

Funding: National Eye Institute, National Institutes of Health.

Year Study Began: 1988.

Year Study Published: 1992.

Study Location: Beaver Dam, Wisconsin, United States.

Who Was Studied: Residents of Beaver Dam. A total of 5,925 adults between the ages of 43 and 84 years were identified by a private phone census; 4,926 agreed to participate and be examined (56% women; 64% in the 75+ age group).

---

* Basic and Clinical Science Course, Section 12. *Retina and Vitreous.* San Francisco: American Academy of Ophthalmology; 2018–2019.

Who Was Excluded: No-one was excluded.

How Many Patients: 4,926 (4,775 with gradable photographs, including 4,514 for both eyes).

Study Overview: The Beaver Dam Eye Study was a population-based cohort study designed to collect information on the prevalence and incidence of age-related cataract, macular degeneration, and diabetic retinopathy.[1-3] The results of the baseline examination for macular degeneration are reported in this paper.[1]

Study Intervention: None—this was a cross-sectional study. Stereoscopic 30° color fundus photographs centered on the disc and macula and a nonstereoscopic color fundus photograph temporal to but including the fovea of each eye were taken. A grid defining 9 subfields was used for grading following a standardized procedure.

Follow-Up: None—this was a cross-sectional study.

Endpoints: Frequency (%), area, and severity, by age group and sex, of drusen, retinal pigment epithelial (RPE) degeneration, retinal pigment and/or neurosensory retinal detachment, subretinal hemorrhage or fibrosis, exudative macular degeneration, and geographic atrophy.

RESULTS

- The prevalence of late age-related maculopathy was 1.6%.
  - Exudative macular degeneration was present in at least 1 eye in 1.2% of the population.
  - Women 75+ years old had a significantly higher frequency of exudative macular degeneration (6.7% vs. 2.6% in men of the same age, $P = .02$).
  - Geographic atrophy was present in at least 1 eye in 0.6% of the population.
- One or more drusen were present in the macular area of at least 1 eye in 95.5% of the population.
  - The largest drusen in an eye was large (> 124 μm) in 1.9% of 43- to 54-year-olds and 24% in persons 75+ years old.
  - There was no difference in sex or laterality in regards to nonexudative macular degeneration.
- People 75 years of age or older had significantly higher frequencies ($P < .01$) of the following characteristics than people 43 to 54 years of

age: larger sized drusen (≥125 μm, 24.0% versus 1.9%), soft indistinct drusen (23.0% versus 2.1%), retinal pigment abnormalities (26.6% versus 7.3%), exudative macular degeneration (5.2% versus 0.1%), and geographic atrophy (2.0% versus 0%).

- Other findings: RPE degeneration in 8.3%, increased retinal pigment in 12.2%, and pigmentary abnormalities (either RPE degeneration or increased retinal pigment) in 13.1%. All 3 findings increased with age.
- A sharp increase in the frequency of pure geographic atrophy was seen in persons 75+ years old.
- The prevalence of any age-related maculopathy increased from 8.5% in people ages 43–54 years to 36.8% in those age 75 years and older.
  - There was no significant difference between the sexes or between right and left eyes.

Criticisms and Limitations: Whether these prevalence estimates can be generalized to the entire US adult population depends on whether the adult population of Beaver Dam, Wisconsin (and in particular the sample examined in this study) is representative of the general US adult population. This cannot be determined, as no sociodemographic or health information is given.

These prevalence rates may slightly underestimate the actual frequencies of macular degeneration because of the higher rates of nonparticipation or ungradable fundus photographs in older people in the study.

Other Relevant Studies and Information:

- The markedly higher prevalence of macular degeneration in people 75 years of age or older is consistent with findings from other studies.[4-9]
- Follow-up of the Beaver Dam cohort showed a 15-year cumulative incidence of 14.3% for early age-related macular degeneration (AMD) (the presence of either soft indistinct drusen or the presence of pigmentary abnormalities together with any type of drusen) and 3.1% for late AMD (presence of exudative AMD or geographic atrophy).[10]
  - The 15-year cumulative incidence of late AMD in people ≥75 years of age was 8%.

Summary and Implications: Signs of age-related maculopathy are common in people 75 years of age or older. Women of this age group have an incidence of exudative macular degeneration 2–3 times higher than their male counterparts.

This study was an early indication that AMD was becoming a public health problem in an aging American population.

CLINICAL CASE: AN ELDERLY COUPLE WITH AGE-RELATED MACULOPATHY

Case History

A heterosexual, white married couple present to your clinic. Both individuals have concerns of progressive blurring of vision. They both state that objects they know to be straight appear curved, but they can still read fine print easily. Both have visual acuities of 20/25 in each eye. They then tell you that an outside eye care provider diagnosed them with macular degeneration, but they wanted your second opinion. After performing a dilated fundus exam, you inform the married couple that you agree with the referring eye care provider. They are curious about their risk of having significant vision loss. According to the Beaver Dam Eye Study, which demographic group is more likely to present with severe disease?

A. Men over 65 years old.
B. Men over 75 years old.
C. Women over 65 years old.
D. Women over 75 years old.

Suggested Answer

The Beaver Dam Eye Study showed that women over the age of 75 years old were more likely to have exudative ARMD (option D).

References

1. Klein R, Klein B, Linton KLP. Prevalence of age-related maculopathy. *Ophthalmology*. 1992;99(6):933–43.
2. Linton KL, Klein BE, Klein R. The validity of self-reported and surrogate-reported cataract and age-related macular degeneration in the Beaver Dam Eye Study. *Am J Epidemiol*. 1991;134(12):1438–46.
3. Klein R, Klein BE, Linton KL, De Mets DL. The Beaver Dam Eye Study: visual acuity. *Ophthalmology*. 1991;98(8):1310–5.
4. Leibowitz HM, Krueger DE, Maunder LR, et al. The Framingham Eye Study Monograph. *Surv Ophthalmol*. 1980;24(Suppl):335–610.

5. Bressler NM, Bressler SB, West SK, Fine SL, Taylor HR. The grading and prevalence of macular degeneration in Chesapeake Bay watermen. *Arch Ophthalmol.* 1989;107(6):847–52.

6. Vingerling JR, Dielemans I, Hofman A, et al. The prevalence of age-related maculopathy in the Rotterdam Study. *Ophthalmology.* 1995;102(2):205–10.

7. Mitchell P, Smith W, Attebo K, Wang JJ. Prevalence of age-related maculopathy in Australia. The Blue Mountains Eye Study. *Ophthalmology.* 1995;102(10):1450–60.

8. Klein R, Clegg L, Cooper LS, et al. Prevalence of age-related maculopathy in the Atherosclerosis Risk in Communities Study. *Arch Ophthalmol.* 1999;117(9):1203–10.

9. VanNewkirk MR, Nanjan MB, Wang JJ, Mitchell P, Taylor HR, McCarty CA. The prevalence of age-related maculopathy: the visual impairment project. *Ophthalmology.* 2000;107(8):1593–600.

10. Klein R, Klein BE, Knudtson MD, Meuer SM, Swift M, Gangnon RE. Fifteen-year cumulative incidence of age-related macular degeneration: the Beaver Dam Eye Study. *Ophthalmology.* 2007;114(2):253–62.

36

Does High-Dose Supplementation with Vitamins C and E, Beta Carotene, and Zinc Slow the Progression of Age-Related Macular Degeneration and Vision Loss?

*Age-Related Eye Disease Study (AREDS)**

[Persons older than 55 years] with extensive intermediate size drusen, at least 1 large druse, noncentral geographic atrophy in 1 or both eyes, or advanced age-related macular degeneration (AMD) or vision loss due to AMD in 1 eye, and without contraindications such as smoking, should consider taking a supplement of antioxidants plus zinc as that used in this study.

—AREDS RESEARCH GROUP[1]

Research Question: What is the effect of high-dose vitamins C and E, beta carotene, and zinc supplements on the progression of age-related macular degeneration (AMD) and vision loss?[1]

Funding: National Eye Institute, National Institutes of Health; Bausch and Lomb Inc. (Rochester, NY).

---

* Basic and Clinical Science Course, Section 12: *Retina and Vitreous.* San Francisco: American Academy of Ophthalmology, 2018–2019: 69–71.

Year Study Began: 1992.

Year Study Published: 2001.

Study Location: 11 retinal specialty clinics.

Who Was Studied: Individuals, 55–80 years of age, were enrolled if they had extensive small drusen, intermediate drusen, large drusen, noncentral geographic atrophy, or pigment abnormalities in 1 or both eyes, or advanced AMD (defined as choroidal neovascularization, other exudative maculopathy, or geographic atrophy involving the center of the macula) or vision loss due to AMD in one eye. At least 1 eye had best corrected visual acuity of 20/32 or better. Participants were classified into 4 categories. Category 2 had multiple small drusen (<63 μm), nonextensive intermediate drusen (63–124 μm), or pigmentary changes. Category 3 had extensive intermediate drusen, any large drusen (≥125 μm), or noncentral geographic atrophy without advanced AMD. Category 4 had advanced AMD in 1 eye but not in the other eye. Persons aged 55 to 59 years were eligible only if they were in Category 3 or 4. (Patients with minimal or no drusen (category 1) were included for concurrent studies of supplementation and cataract.)

Who Was Excluded: Individuals were not enrolled unless the ocular media were sufficiently clear to obtain adequate quality stereoscopic fundus photographs of the macula. At least 1 eye of each participant had to be free from any eye disease that could complicate assessment of AMD, lens opacity progression, or visual acuity (e.g., optic atrophy, acute uveitis), and that eye could not have had previous ocular surgery (other than cataract surgery).

How Many Patients: 3,640 in the AMD trial.

Study Overview: AREDS was a randomized, double-masked clinical trial with 2 components, an AMD trial and a cataract trial (Figure 36.1).[1,2]

Study Intervention: Participants were randomly assigned to receive daily oral tablets containing: (1) antioxidants (vitamin C, 500 mg; vitamin E, 400 IU; and beta carotene, 15 mg); (2) zinc, 80 mg, as zinc oxide, and copper, 2 mg, as cupric oxide; (3) antioxidants plus zinc; or (4) placebo. Two study medication tablets were to be taken each morning and 2 each evening to meet the total daily dose requirement.

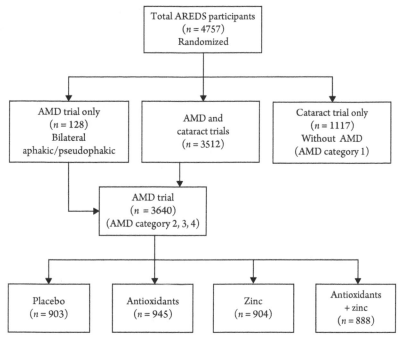

Figure 36.1 Summary of AREDS.

Follow-Up: Average follow-up was 6.3 years.

Endpoints: (1) Photographic assessment of progression to, or treatment for, advanced AMD and (2) at least moderate visual acuity loss from baseline (≥ 15 letters).

RESULTS

- At 5 years, the estimated probability of progression to advanced AMD was 28% for those assigned to placebo; 23% and 22% for those assigned to antioxidants and zinc, respectively; and 20% for those assigned to antioxidants plus zinc.
- Comparison with placebo demonstrated a statistically significant odds reduction for the development of advanced AMD with antioxidants plus zinc (odds ratio [OR], 0.72).
  - The ORs for zinc alone and antioxidants alone were 0.75 and 0.80, respectively.
- Participants with extensive small drusen, nonextensive intermediate size drusen, or pigment abnormalities (category 2) had only a 1.3% 5-year probability of progression to advanced AMD.

- Odds reduction estimates increased when the analysis was restricted to participants in categories 3 and 4: antioxidants plus zinc: OR= 0.66; zinc: OR = 0.71; antioxidants: OR = 0.76.
- Both zinc and antioxidants plus zinc significantly reduced the odds of developing advanced AMD in this higher-risk group.
- The only statistically significant reduction in rates of at least moderate visual acuity loss occurred in persons assigned to receive antioxidants plus zinc (OR, 0.73).
- No statistically significant serious adverse effect was associated with any of the formulations.
- Category 2 participants had only a 1.3% probability of progression to advanced AMD by year 5, but Category 3 had an 18% probability of progression. Within the Category 3 group, half of the participants had large drusen in each eye or noncentral geographic atrophy in at least 1 eye at enrollment, and these participants were 4 times as likely to progress to advanced AMD compared with the remaining Category 3 participants. The Category 4 group had a 43% expected probability of progression to advanced AMD in the fellow study eye at 5 years.
- At 5 years, the estimated probability of at least a 15-letter decrease in visual acuity score from baseline was 29% for those assigned to placebo, 26% for those assigned to antioxidants, 25% for those assigned to zinc, and 23% for those assigned to antioxidants plus zinc.

Criticisms and Limitations: While the results of the study were statistically significant, the clinical impact of AREDS supplementation in reducing the progression to late AMD is modest. There is some question whether the AREDS findings were generalizable to other populations with different nutritional statuses. The study also did not address differing doses of supplementation, which are relevant considering past data concerning long-term harm from supplementation. Long-term safety information was lacking regarding supplementation.

Other Relevant Studies and Information:

- The AREDS2 research group was later established to evaluate the addition of lutein/zeaxanthin and omega-3 long-chain polyunsaturated fatty acids to the original AREDS.[2] Modifications to the original study included elimination of beta carotene and reduction of zinc level to 25 mg. Participants were restricted to those with bilateral large drusen or late AMD in 1 eye. The study noted no significant effect with omega-3 fatty acids and that the combination of lutein and zeaxanthin had an incremental beneficial effect. The substitution of lutein and zeaxanthin for beta carotene was necessary given that beta carotene was found to increase the risk of lung cancer 2-fold, especially in former smokers.

- New data regarding the genetic associations with AMD have peaked interest in how certain variants may influence AREDS supplementation. Klein et al found that some differences may exist between AMD genetic variants and response to AREDS but that all subjects, regardless of genotype, responded to AREDS supplements.[3] The study proposed that no genetic testing should be done prior to initiating AREDS supplementation due to this overall positive response.

Summary and Implications: Individuals aged 55 years and older should have dilated eye examinations to determine their risk of developing advanced AMD. Those with extensive intermediate size drusen, at least 1 large druse, noncentral geographic atrophy in 1 or both eyes, or advanced AMD or vision loss due to AMD in 1 eye, and without contraindications such as smoking, should consider taking a supplement of antioxidants (consisting of vitamin C and E and beta carotene) plus zinc. Based on this study, additional studies led to a change in the formula for the AREDS vitamins (beta carotene was replaced with lutein and zeaxanthin in a formula called "AREDS2"), but the recommendation to take daily supplementation still stands for patients who have fundus exam findings consistent with Category 3 or worse.

CLINICAL CASE: A MIDDLE-AGED WOMAN WITH AMD

Case History

A 55-year-old Caucasian woman presents to your clinic with a chief complaint of decreased vision. Upon examination, visual acuities are 20/25 in the right eye and 20/60 in the left eye. Fundus exam shows extensive intermediate drusen of both eyes with noncentral geographic atrophy involving only 1 eye. After discussing lifestyle changes to decrease her probability of progression, she asks you if there is any "pill or eyedrop" she could take that would decrease her chances of progression. What do you recommend to the patient as the best treatment option for her to minimize her chances of progressing to advanced AMD?

A. Observation only.
B. Antioxidants (vitamin C and E, beta carotene).
C. Zinc.
D. Antioxidants plus zinc.

Suggested Answer

The examination findings in this patient are typical for "dry" AMD corresponding to Category 3 of the AREDS study. Based on the results of report 8 of the AREDS study, she should be advised to take the AREDS vitamin formulation including antioxidants plus zinc (option D) to decrease her risk of progressing to advanced AMD.

References

1. Age-Related Eye Disease Study Group. A randomized, placebo-controlled clinical trial of high-dose supplementation with vitamins C and E, beta carotene, and zinc for age-related macular degeneration and vision loss: AREDS report no. 8. *Arch Ophthalmol.* 2001;119(10):1417–36.
2. Age-Related Eye Disease Study 2 Research Group. Lutein + zeaxanthin and omega-3 fatty acids for age-related macular degeneration: the Age-Related Eye Disease Study 2 Research group. *JAMA.*2013;309(19):2005–2015.
3. Klein ML, Francis PJ, Rosner B, et al. CFH and LOC387715/ARMS2 genotypes and treatment with antioxidants and zinc for age-related macular degeneration. *Ophthalmology.* 2008;115(6):1019–1025.

37

Argon Laser Photocoagulation for Extrafoveal Neovascular Maculopathy*

Macular Photocoagulation Study

[It is recommended that] eyes with well-defined extrafoveal choroidal neovascular membranes secondary to senile macular degeneration, ocular histoplasmosis, and idiopathic causes be treated with argon laser photocoagulation.

— MACULAR PHOTOCOAGULATION STUDY GROUP[1]

Research Question: Does coagulating a leaking blood vessel outside the fovea prevent significant loss of visual acuity?[1]

Funding: National Eye Institute, National Institutes of Health.

Year Study Began: 1979.

Year Study Published: 1990.

Study Location: 12 centers in the United States.

Who Was Studied: Patients, 50 years of age and older, were eligible if they had: (1) ophthalmoscopic evidence of macular degeneration, histoplasmosis,

* Basic and Clinical Science Course, Section 12: Retina and Vitreous. San Francisco: American Academy of Ophthalmology, 2018–2019.

or idiopathic choroidal neovascularization; (2) angiographic evidence of choroidal neovascularization outside the fovea (200 to 2,500 μm from center of
the foveal avascular zone [FAZ]); (3) best corrected visual acuity of 20/100 or
better in the eye to be entered; (4) symptoms related to neovascular membrane,
e.g., decreased acuity, Amsler grid distortion, metamorphopsia, or uniocular diplopia. Eyes with peripapillary membranes were included only if the photocoagulation required to cover the neovascular complex would spare at least 1 ½ clock
hours of the peripapillary nerve fiber layer adjacent to the disc.

Who Was Excluded: Patients were excluded if they had had prior photocoagulation in the study eye or other ocular disease that could independently affect
visual acuity.

How Many Patients: 565.

Study Overview: The Macular Photocoagulation Study (MPS) comprised three
randomized clinical trials: the Senile Macular Degeneration Study (SMDS), the
Ocular Histoplasmosis Study (OHS), and the Idiopathic Neovascularization
Study (INVS) (Figure 37.1).[1,2]

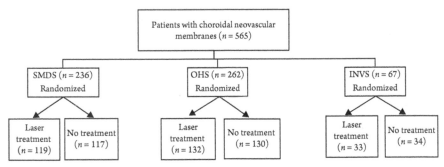

Figure 37.1 Summary of the Macular Photocoagulation study.

Study Intervention: Treatment was performed using 200-μm spots of 0.5-sec. duration at a sufficient intensity to produce a uniformly white lesion that extended beyond the neovascular complex by 100 to 125 μm on all sides. For neovascular lesions
within 350 μm of the center of the FAZ, 100-μm spots of 0.2-sec. duration were used
to coagulate along the foveal perimeter of the neovascularization. The goal of treatment was to obliterate the neovascular complex completely. Therefore, coagulations
were extended 100 to 125 μm beyond any adjacent blood, pigmentation, or blocked
fluorescence so that any occult neovascularization would be treated.

Follow-Up: 5 years.

Endpoints: Best corrected visual acuity.

RESULTS

- In eyes with senile (age-related) macular degeneration, the relative risk of losing six or more lines of visual acuity from the baseline level among untreated eyes compared with laser-treated eyes was 1.5 from 6 months through 5 years after entry ($P = .001$).
    - After 5 years, untreated eyes had lost a mean of 7.1 lines of visual acuity, while laser-treated eyes had lost 5.2 lines.
    - Recurrent neovascularization had been observed in 54% of laser-treated eyes by the end of the 5-year follow-up period.
    - Nearly 80% of eyes that experienced recurrence were observed to do so within 1 year after initial treatment.
- Among eyes with ocular histoplasmosis, untreated eyes had 3.6 times the risk of laser-treated eyes of losing 6 or more lines of visual acuity ($P < .0001$).
    - Untreated eyes had lost a mean of 4.4 lines of visual acuity after 5 years, compared with only 0.9 lines lost by laser-treated eyes.
    - Among laser-treated eyes, recurrent neovascularization had been observed in 26% by 5 years after enrollment.
- When the extrafoveal lesion was due to idiopathic causes, the relative risk of losing 6 or more lines of visual acuity from the baseline level among untreated eyes compared with laser-treated eyes was 2.3 ($P = .04$).
    - The mean number of lines of visual acuity lost from baseline to the 5-year examination was 4.4 among untreated eyes and 2.7 among laser-treated eyes.
    - Recurrent neovascularization was observed in 34% of laser-treated eyes during 5 years of follow-up.
- Generally, recurrence was accompanied by an increased frequency of severe visual loss.
    - It was not possible to accurately predict recurrence.
    - Cigarette smoking was related to the rate of recurrence in the SMDS ($P = .02$) and the INVS ($P = .09$). Younger age and female gender were associated with an increased frequency of recurrence in the OHS.

Criticisms and Limitations: The results do not apply to asymptomatic eyes, to eyes with drusen without a neovascular membrane, or to eyes with geographic retinal pigment epithelial (RPE) atrophy, serous or hemorrhagic detachments of the RPE, fibrous disciform scars, or neovascular membranes within 200 μm of the center of the FAZ.

Most patients referred for possible enrollment in the MPS were not eligible for treatment according to the MPS angiographic criteria. The authors reported that often it was necessary to screen 20 or more patients with SMD with visual loss caused by exudative maculopathy to find a single patient who met the eligibility criteria.

Other Relevant Studies and Information:

- The MPS also conducted a parallel series of 3 randomized clinical trials of krypton red laser treatment of juxtafoveal neovascular lesions (choroidal neovascularization 1 to 199 microns from the center of the FAZ or choroidal neovascularization 200 microns or further from the FAZ center with blood and pigment extending within 200 microns of the FAZ center) secondary to age-related macular degeneration (AMD), ocular histoplasmosis, or idiopathic causes. The early beneficial effects of laser treatment on visual acuity persisted for at least 5 years in eyes with all three underlying conditions. Laser treatment of similar eyes with choroidal neovascularization in a juxtafoveal location was recommended for patients with these conditions, with the caveat that hypertensive patients with AMD may fare no better with laser treatment than without treatment.[4]

Summary and Implications: Patients with visual symptoms due to well-defined extrafoveal choroidal neovascular membranes (at least 200 microns from the center of the FAZ) and a best corrected visual acuity of 20/100 or better secondary to senile macular degeneration, ocular histoplasmosis, and idiopathic causes should be treated with argon blue-green laser photocoagulation to prevent or delay significant loss of visual acuity. Careful follow-up of all treated eyes is indicated, particularly within the first year after initial argon photocoagulation.

CLINICAL CASE: AN ELDERLY PATIENT WITH CNVM

Case History
An elderly patient presents with decreased acuity and metamorphopsia in one eye, and is found to have a well-defined extrafoveal choroidal neovascular membrane (CNVM) of uncertain etiology . In the absence of access to any more modern treatments, such as anti–vascular endothelial growth factor injections, you recommend treatment with argon laser photocoagulation.

According to the Macular Photocoagulation Study Group, which of the following statements is true for the prevention or delay of severe loss of visual acuity in this situation?

A. In patients with extrafoveal CNVM at least 100 microns from the center of the FAZ secondary to senile macular degeneration, argon blue-green laser treatment was demonstrated to be significantly better than observation only to prevent or delay significant loss of visual acuity.
B. In patients with extrafoveal CNVM secondary to ocular histoplasmosis, argon blue-green laser treatment was demonstrated to be worse than observation only to prevent or delay significant loss of visual acuity..
C. In patients with extrafoveal CNVM secondary to idiopathic causes, argon blue-green laser treatment was demonstrated to be no better than observation only to prevent or delay significant loss of visual acuity.
D. In patients with extrafoveal CNVM at least 200 microns from center of the FAZ secondary to senile macular degeneration, ocular histoplasmosis, or idiopathic causes, argon blue-green laser treatment was demonstrated to be significantly better than observation only to prevent or delay significant loss of visual acuity.

Suggested Answer
Option D. At the time of publication, the Macular Photocoagulation Study Group rrecommended that symptomatic eyes with well-defined extrafoveal choroidal neovascular membranes (at least 200 microns from center of the FAZ) secondary to senile macular degeneration, ocular histoplasmosis, and idiopathic causes be treated with argon blue-green laser photocoagulation.

References

1. Argon laser photocoagulation for neovascular maculopathy. Five-year results from randomized clinical trials. Macular Photocoagulation Study Group. *Arch Ophthalmol.* 1991;109(8):1109–14.
2. Argon laser photocoagulation for senile macular degeneration. Results of a randomized clinical trial. *Arch Ophthalmol.* 1982;100(6):912–8.
3. Recurrent choroidal neovascularization after argon laser photocoagulation for neovascular maculopathy. Macular Photocoagulation Study Group. *Arch Ophthalmol.* 1986;104(4):503–12.
4. Laser photocoagulation for juxtafoveal choroidal neovascularization. Five-year results from randomized clinical trials. Macular Photocoagulation Study Group. *Arch Ophthalmol.* 1994;112(4):500–9.

38

Photodynamic Therapy of Subfoveal Choroidal Neovascularization in Age-Related Macular Degeneration with Verteporfin[*]

Treatment of Age-Related Macular Degeneration with Photodynamic Therapy (TAP) Study

> Since verteporfin therapy of subfoveal CNV from AMD can safely reduce the risk of vision loss, we recommend verteporfin therapy for treatment of patients with predominantly classic CNV from AMD.
>
> —TAP STUDY GROUP[1]

Research Question: Does photodynamic treatment with verteporfin reduce the risk of vision loss in patients with age-related macular degeneration (AMD) due to subfoveal choroidal neovascularization (CNV)?[1]

Funding: QLT PhotoTherapeutics Inc., Canada; CIBA Vision AG, Switzerland.

Year Study Began: 1996.

Year Study Published: 1999.

Study Location: 22 ophthalmology practices in Europe and North America.

[*] Basic and Clinical Science Course, Section 12. *Retina and Vitreous*. San Francisco: American Academy of Ophthalmology; 2018–2019: 380.

Who Was Studied: Patients 50 years of age or older with evidence of classic CNV secondary to AMD located under the geometric center of the foveal avascular zone. The area of CNV had to be at least 50% of the area of the total neovascular lesion, and the lesion had to be smaller than 5400 μm in its greatest linear dimension. The patient's best corrected vision had to be between 20/40 and 20/200 Snellen equivalent.

Who Was Excluded: Patients were excluded if they had a tear in the retinal pigment epithelium, any significant ocular disease (other than CNV) or recent ocular surgery, prior photodynamic therapy (PDT) for CNV or any history of treatment for CNV other than nonfoveal confluent laser photocoagulation, active hepatitis, significant liver disease, or porphyria/porphyrin sensitivity.

How Many Patients: 609.

Study Overview: The TAP Report 1 details 1-year results of 2, double-masked, placebo-controlled, randomized clinical trials (Figure 38.1).[1,2]

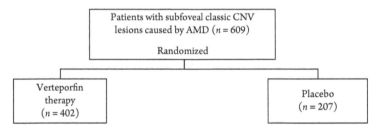

Figure 38.1 Summary of the TAP study.

Study Intervention: Patients were randomly allocated to receive verteporfin therapy or placebo (2:1 verteporfin to placebo randomization). The verteporfin group was given an intravenous infusion of 30 mL verteporfin (a photosensitizer) over 10 minutes, followed by a laser light at 689 nm over 83 seconds, starting at 15 minutes after the start of the infusion; the placebo group received 30 mL intravenous 5% dextrose in water over 10 minutes followed by the same laser therapy at 15 minutes. Retreatment with the same regimen was performed every 3 months if angiography showed fluorescein leakage.

Follow-Up: 12 months.

Endpoints: The primary outcome was the proportion of eyes with fewer than 15 letters lost (approximately <3 lines).

RESULTS

- Visual acuity, contrast sensitivity, and fluorescein angiographic outcomes were better in the verteporfin-treated eyes than in the placebo-treated eyes at every follow-up examination (starting at month 3) through the month 12 examination.
- At the 12-month exam, 61% of eyes treated with verteporfin lost fewer than 15 letters of visual acuity from baseline, whereas 46% assigned to placebo lost fewer than 15 letters ($P <.001$)
  - When the area of classic CNV occupied >50% of the entire lesion, the benefit of verteporfin therapy was more pronounced (67% verteporfin treated had <15 letters lost vs. 39% in the placebo group, $P < .001$).
  - No statistically significant difference was found when the area of classic CNV was <50% of the total area of the lesion.
- Although both groups had a similar mean visual acuity at baseline (approximate Snellen equivalent of 20/80–2), by month 12 the mean visual acuity in eyes treated with verteporfin compared with eyes given placebo was 20/160+2 vs. 20/200.
- Fluorescein angiographic assessments at follow-up examinations suggested that verteporfin treatment reduced lesion growth, was associated with cessation of leakage from classic CNV, and decreased the progression of classic CNV.
- Few ocular or other systemic adverse events were associated with verteporfin treatment, compared with placebo, including transient visual disturbances (18% vs. 12%), injection-site adverse events (13% vs. 3%), transient photosensitivity reactions (3% vs. 0%), and infusion-related low back pain (2% vs. 0%).

Criticisms and Limitations: Initial criticisms of this trial included discussion about how well clinicians could differentiate classic CNV lesions from their occult counterparts, since the trial suggested that only predominantly classic CNV lesions benefited from verteporfin therapy.[3] The cost-effectiveness of verteporfin therapy was also analyzed given the frequency of follow-up, testing, and treatment, and the moderate amount of vision preservation compared to placebo at 1 year. The treatment was initially said to be cost-ineffective given the 2-year results.[4] However, this was disputed at the conclusion of the 5-year study and debated further in later publications.[5,6]

This trial did not investigate patients with CNV lesions larger than 5400 μm or lesions that were not located in the geometric center of the foveal avascular zone, therefore limiting the external validity of the study to those patients with these particular findings.

Other Relevant Studies and Information:

- During the second year of follow-up of the TAP Study cohort, the same regimen (with verteporfin or placebo as applied at baseline) was used if angiography showed fluorescein leakage from CNV. Beneficial outcomes with respect to visual acuity and contrast sensitivity noted at the month 12 examination in verteporfin-treated patients were sustained through the month 24 examination.
  - At month 24, 213 (53%) of 402 verteporfin-treated patients compared with 78 (38%) of 207 placebo-treated patients lost fewer than 15 letters ($P < .001$).
  - In participants with predominantly classic lesions (in which the area of classic CNV makes up at least 50% of the area of the entire lesion) at baseline, 94 (59%) of 159 verteporfin-treated patients compared with 26 (31%) of 83 placebo-treated patients lost fewer than 15 letters at the month 24 examination ($P <.001$).
  - For minimally classic lesions (in which the area of classic CNV makes up <50% but >0% of the area of the entire lesion) at baseline, no statistically significant differences in visual acuity were noted.[7]
- Of the 402 verteporfin-treated patients in the randomized trials, 320 (80%) enrolled in the extension study; 193 (60%) of these completed the extension study up to 5 years.[8] Vision outcomes remained relatively stable from month 24 to month 60 even though the treatment rate was low during this period.
  - Seventy-seven (62%) of the 124 verteporfin-treated patients with predominantly classic lesions at baseline who enrolled in the extension completed the month 60 examination. Twenty-six (34%) of these 77 patients had lost 3 or more lines of visual acuity by month 24 and 27 (35%) had lost this amount of vision by month 60; the mean change in visual acuity from baseline was also similar at the month 24 and month 60 examinations (-1.5 and -1.6 lines, respectively).
- A companion study, called the Verteporfin in Photodynamic Therapy (VIP) Trial, was also carried out during this same time period, and included patients that were excluded from the TAP trial. These patients had evidence of occult CNV without classic CNV. The results of this trial suggested a benefit in this patient group as well, especially when the lesion was small in size.[9]

- By month 24, the verteporfin-treated eyes were less likely to have moderate or severe vision loss. Of the 225 verteporfin-treated patients, 121 (54%) compared with 76 (67%) of 114 placebo-treated patients lost at least 15 letters (P =.023). Likewise, 67 of the verteporfin-treated patients (30%) compared with 54 of the placebo-treated patients (47%) lost at least 30 letters (P =.001).
- In a 2-year study comparing ranibizumab with verteporfin photodynamic therapy (PDT) in treating predominantly classic CNV, ranibizumab provided greater clinical benefit than verteporfin PDT in patients with AMD with new-onset, predominantly classic CNV, with low rates of serious adverse events.[10]
- Currently, anti-VEGF agents are first-line therapy for treating neovascular AMD; however, PDT can be useful in patients with refractory AMD when anti-VEGF monotherapy options have been exhausted.[11]

Summary and Implications: Photodynamic therapy with verteporfin safely reduces the chance of vision loss in patients who have AMD with predominantly classic subfoveal choroidal neovascularization.

CLINICAL CASE: AN ELDERLY WOMAN WITH CNV SECONDARY TO AMD

Case History

A 73-year-old white woman presents to your clinic complaining of blurred vision in the right eye for the past 3 weeks. She has never experienced anything like this before, and states that she cannot seem to focus on anything in her central vision, but sees everything in the peripheral vision clearly.

On examination her visual acuity is 20/200 in the right eye and 20/25 in the left eye. She has no relative afferent pupillary defect. Intraocular pressure is within normal limits and the anterior segment examination is largely unremarkable. The fundus exam reveals numerous drusen in both eyes and macular edema in the right eye. According to the TAP study, which description of choroidal neovascularization seen on fluorescein angiography would benefit from photodynamic therapy with verteporfin in this patient?

A. a 6000 μm subfoveal occult CNV lesion.
B. a 4800 μm subfoveal classic CNV lesion.

C. a 5000 μm fovea-sparing classic CNV lesion.

D. a 4200 μm subfoveal occult CNV lesion.

Suggested Answer

The history and examination findings in this patient are suggestive of AMD with exudative transformation in the right eye. Based on the results of the TAP study, only classic, subfoveal CNV lesions less than 5400 μm across showed a benefit from photodynamic therapy with verteporfin (option B).

References

1. Treatment of Age-Related Macular Degeneration With Photodynamic Therapy (TAP) Study Group. Photodynamic therapy of subfoveal choroidal neovascularization in age-related macular degeneration with verteporfin: one-year results of 2 randomized clinical trials- TAP Report 1. *Arch Ophthalmol.* 1999;117(10):1329–45.

2. Mones J, for the VIP Study Group, Photodynamic therapy (PDT) with verteporfin of the subfoveal choroidal neovascularization in age-related macular degeneration: study design and baseline characteristics in the VIP randomized clinical trial. *Invest Opthalmol Vis Sci.* 1999;40:S321.

3. Fine SL. Photodynamic therapy with verteporfin is effective for selected patients with neovascular age-related macular degeneration. *Arch Ophthalmol.* 1999;117(10):1400–2.

4. Sharma S Sharma S, Brown GC, Brown MM, Hollands H, Shah GK. The cost-effectiveness of photodynamic therapy for fellow eyes with subfoveal choroidal neovascularization secondary to age-related macular degeneration. *Ophthalmology.* 2001;108(11):2051–9.

5. Brown GC, Brown MM, Campanella J, Beauchamp GR. The cost-utility of photodynamic therapy in eyes with neovascular macular degeneration: a value-based reappraisal with 5-year data. *Am J Ophthalmol.* 2005; 140(4):679–87.

6. Grieve R, Guerriero C, Walker J, et al.; Verteporfin Photodynamic Therapy Cohort Study Group. Verteporfin Photodynamic Therapy Cohort Study: Report 3: cost effectiveness and lessons for future evaluations. *Ophthalmology.* 2009;116(12):2471–7.

7. Bressler NM; Treatment of Age-Related Macular Degeneration with Photodynamic Therapy (TAP) Study Group. Photodynamic therapy of subfoveal choroidal neovascularization in age-related macular degeneration with verteporfin: two-year results of 2 randomized clinical trials-tap report 2. *Arch Ophthalmol.* 2001;119(2):198–207.

8. Kaiser PK. Verteporfin therapy of subfoveal choroidal neovascularization in age-related macular degeneration: 5-year results of two randomized clinical trials with an open-label extension. TAP Report No. 8. *Graefes Arch Clin Exp Ophthalmol.* 2006;244(9):1132–42.

9. Verteporfin in Photodynamic Therapy Study Group. Verteporfin therapy of subfoveal choroidal neovascularization in age-related macular degeneration: two-year results of a randomized clinical trial including lesions with occult with no classic choroidal

neovascularization--verteporfin in photodynamic therapy report 2. *Am J Ophthalmol.* 2001;131(5):541–60.

10. Brown DM, Michels M, Kaiser PK, Heier JS, Sy JP, Ianchulev T; ANCHOR Study Group. Ranibizumab versus verteporfin photodynamic therapy for neovascular age-related macular degeneration: Two-year results of the ANCHOR study. *Ophthalmology.* 2009;116(1):57–65.e5.

11. Fernandez-Robredo P, Sancho A, Johnen S, et al. Current treatment limitations in age-related macular degeneration and future approaches based on cell therapy and tissue engineering. *J Ophthalmol.* 2014;20:510285.

39

Pegaptanib for Neovascular Age-Related Macular Degeneration*

VEGF Inhibition Study in Ocular Neovascularization (V.I.S.I.O.N.) Clinical Trial

Continuing visual benefit was observed in patients who were random-ized to receive therapy with pegaptanib in year 2 of the V.I.S.I.O.N. trials when compared with 2 years' usual care or cessation of therapy at year 1.
—V.I.S.I.O.N. STUDY GROUP[1]

Research Question: To evaluate the efficacy and safety of a second year of pegaptanib sodium therapy in patients with neovascular age-related macular degeneration (AMD).[1]

Funding: Eyetech Pharmaceuticals, Inc., New York; Pfizer Inc., New York.

Year Study Began: 2001.

Year Study Published: 2006.

Study Location: 117 sites in the United States, Canada, Europe, Israel, Australia, and South America.

Who Was Studied: Patients 50 years of age or older with subfoveal choroidal neovascularization secondary to AMD and a best corrected visual acuity (VA)

* Basic and Clinical Science Course, Section 12. *Retina and Vitreous.* San Francisco: American Academy of Ophthalmology; 2018–2019: 80, 87.

of 20/40 to 20/320 in the study eye and 20/800 or better in the other eye. To avoid enrollment of totally quiescent or involuted occult lesions, documented evidence of a 15-letter loss in the 12 weeks before enrollment was one of the criteria. Patients with a history of up to 1 previous administration of photodynamic therapy with verteporfin were eligible provided administration was within 8 to 13 weeks before enrollment.

Who Was Excluded: Patients with VA worse than 20/800 in the fellow eye were not eligible, as were those with lesion size exceeding 12 disc areas, <50% of the lesion having active choroidal neovascularization, and hemorrhage accounting for >50% of the lesion. Lesions could comprise up to 25% scars or atrophy but could not contain any subfoveal scars or atrophy. Patients with <50% classic lesion composition were required to have either subretinal hemorrhage (comprising up to 50% of the lesion) and/or documented evidence of ≥3 lines' vision loss in the 12 weeks before baseline and/or lipid.

How Many Patients: 1,190.

Study Overview: The VEGF Inhibition Study in Ocular Neovascularization comprised two concurrent randomized, double-masked, sham-controlled studies (Figure 39.1).[1,2]

Study Intervention: In the initial study, patients were randomly assigned to receive either sham injection or intravitreous injection of pegaptanib into one eye every 6 weeks over a period of 48 weeks, for a total of 9 treatments. To maintain masking of the patients, the patients receiving sham injections and those receiving the study medication were treated identically, with the exception of scleral penetration.

At week 54, those initially assigned to pegaptanib were rerandomized (1:1) to continue or discontinue therapy for 48 more weeks (8 injections). Those initially assigned to sham were rerandomized to continue sham, discontinue sham, or receive 1 of 3 pegaptanib doses. Rescue therapy was allowed during the second year in those rerandomized to stop treatment at week 54. Eighty-eight percent (1053/1190) of patients who received at least 1 treatment during the first year of the study were rerandomized at week 54; 89% (941/1053) of patients rerandomized at week 54 were assessed at week 102.

Follow-Up: 2 years (102 weeks).

Endpoints: Year 2 efficacy end points included the mean change in VA over time from week 54 to week 102 and Kaplan-Meier proportions of the loss of an

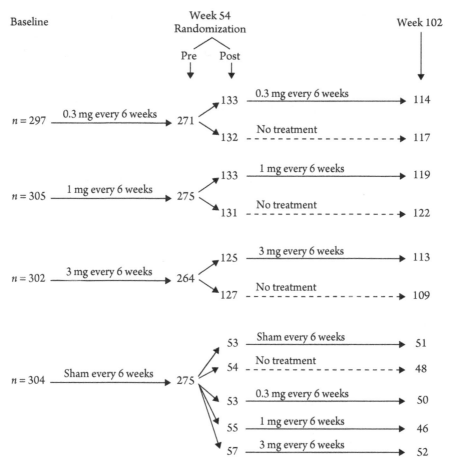

Figure 39.1 Summary of V.I.S.I.O.N.

additional 15 letters of vision from week 54 to week 102 (comparing patients who continued with active therapy with those who discontinued).

RESULTS

- In the combined analysis, the mean VA of patients continuing with 0.3 mg pegaptanib remained stable during the second year of therapy, compared with those discontinuing therapy or receiving usual care.
  - Mean VA decreased in patients rerandomized to stop pegaptanib after 1 year of therapy.
  - VA also decreased in those who received usual care continuously from baseline and this group had the poorest visual outcome.

- In patients who continued pegaptanib, the proportion who lost >15 letters from baseline in the period from week 54 to week 102 was half (7%) that of patients who discontinued pegaptanib or remained on usual care (14% for each).
- The proportion of patients gaining vision was higher for those assigned to 2 years of 0.3-mg pegaptanib than receiving usual care.
- Patients in the pegaptanib group had lower rates of progression to legal blindness in the second year of the study than those who were randomized to discontinue therapy and those who received usual care from baseline.
- Although patients randomized to discontinue pegaptanib were at a greater risk of vision loss than those continuing with therapy, the results demonstrated that vision loss after discontinuation did not exceed the rate expected by natural history—that is, there was no rebound effect due to discontinuation.
- There was no evidence that concomitant treatment with photodynamic therapy, which was allowed at the investigators' discretion, confounded the results.

Criticisms and Limitations: The trials were not designed to identify whether patients with particular baseline characteristics (such as baseline VA and/or lesion type/size) might experience enhanced or diminished benefit from 2 years' continuous vascular endothelial growth factor (VEGF) inhibition with pegaptanib.

It is possible that the outcomes at week 102 for patients discontinuing therapy at year 1 might have been inflated by random imbalances at the week 54 rerandomization and by rescue treatments, thereby underestimating the importance of continued treatment for 2 years. (After rerandomization at week 54, patients continuing 0.3-mg pegaptanib had a 44-letter mean VA [approximately 20/125 Snellen equivalent] compared to a 50-letter mean VA [approximately 20/100 Snellen equivalent] in those discontinuing pegaptanib.)

There is also a likelihood that rescue therapy given to a sizable proportion of patients during year 2 and the subsequent protection through the potential avoidance of a 3-line loss from baseline to week 102 contributed to a further underestimation of the value of treatment. Kaplan-Meier curves were selected as an alternative analysis for this reason.

Other Relevant Studies and Information:

- A separate study to evaluate the safety of pegaptanib sodium injection reported that all doses of pegaptanib were well tolerated and that the 2-year safety profile was favorable.[3]

- The most common ocular adverse events were transient, mild to moderate in intensity, and attributed to the injection preparation and procedure. There was no evidence of an increase in deaths, in events associated with systemic VEGF inhibition (e.g., hypertension, thromboembolic events, serious hemorrhagic events), or in severe ocular inflammation, cataract progression, or glaucoma in pegaptanib-treated patients relative to sham-treated patients.
- In year 1, serious injection-related complications included endophthalmitis (12 events, 0.16%/injection), retinal detachment (RD) (6 events [4 rhegmatogenous, 2 exudative], 0.08%/injection), and traumatic cataract (5 events, 0.07%/injection). Most cases of endophthalmitis followed violations of the injection preparation protocol. In patients receiving pegaptanib for >1 year, there were no reports of endophthalmitis or traumatic cataract in year 2; RD was reported in 4 patients (all rhegmatogenous, 0.15%/injection).
- A systematic review of the clinical effectiveness and cost-effectiveness of ranibizumab and pegaptanib for subfoveal choroidal neovascularization associated with "wet" AMD confirmed that patients with AMD of any lesion type benefit from treatment with pegaptanib or ranibizumab on measures of visual acuity when compared with sham injection and/or photodynamic therapy. Patients who continued treatment with either drug appeared to maintain benefits after 2 years of follow-up.[4]

Summary and Implications: In patients with a diverse mix of neovascular AMD presentations, treatment with pegaptanib every 6 weeks for 2 years reduced the risk of vision loss regardless of lesion composition or size; this benefit was maintained during year 2. The data suggest that VEGF is important throughout the evolution of active neovascular AMD.

CLINICAL CASE: AN ELDERLY WOMAN WITH "WET" AMD

Case History

A 65-year-old white woman presents to your clinic with complaints of metamorphopsia for a few weeks in the right eye with a best corrected VA of 20/60. Exam is suggestive of wet ARMD. This is confirmed by optical coherence tomography and fluorescein angiography, which show a subfoveal choroidal neovascular membrane (CNVM). Based on the results of the V.I.S.I.O.N. trial, which treatment protocol would provide the most benefit to the patient?

A. Observation only.
B. Photodyamic therapy with verteporforin.
C. Pegaptanib 0.3% intravitreal injection and re-evaluation and likely repeat injection in 6 weeks.
D. Pegaptanib 0.3% intravitreal injection and re-evaluation and likely repeat injection in 12 weeks.

Suggested Answer

In the V.I.S.I.O.N. study, pegaptanib given every 6 weeks showed significant benefit compared to no treatment (option C). Subsequent systematic review has confirmed that treatment with pegaptanib or ranibizumab has beneficial effects on measures of visual acuity when compared with photodynamic therapy.

References

1. VEGF Inhibition Study in Ocular Neovascularization (V.I.S.I.O.N.) Clinical Trial Group, Chakravarthy U, Adamis AP, Cunningham ET Jr, et al. Year 2 efficacy results of 2 randomized controlled clinical trials of pegaptanib for neovascular age-related macular degeneration. *Ophthalmology*. 2006;113(9):1508.e1–25.
2. Gragoudas ES, Adamis AP, Cunningham ET Jr, Feinsod M, Guyer DR; VEGF Inhibition Study in Ocular Neovascularization Clinical Trial Group. Pegaptanib for neovascular age-related macular degeneration. *N Engl J Med*. 2004;351(27):2805–16.
3. VEGF Inhibition Study in Ocular Neovascularization (V.I.S.I.O.N.) Clinical Trial Group, D'Amico DJ, Masonson HN, Patel M, et al. Pegaptanib sodium for neovascular age-related macular degeneration: two-year safety results of the two prospective, multicenter, controlled clinical trials. *Ophthalmology*. 2006;113(6):992–1001.e6.
4. Colquitt JL, Jones J, Tan SC, Takeda A, Clegg AJ, Price A. Ranibizumab and pegaptanib for the treatment of age-related macular degeneration: a systematic review and economic evaluation. *Health Technol Assess*. 2008;12(16):ii–iv, ix–201.

40

Ranibizumab for Neovascular Age-Related Macular Degeneration[*]

Minimally Classic/Occult Trial of the Anti-VEGF Antibody Ranibizumab in the Treatment of Neovascular AMD (MARINA)

Intravitreal administration of ranibizumab for 2 years prevented vision loss and improved mean visual acuity, with low rates of serious adverse events, in patients with minimally classic or occult (with no classic lesions) choroidal neovascularization secondary to age-related macular degeneration.

—MARINA Study Group[1]

Research Question: Can intravitreal administration of ranibizumab prevent vision loss and improve mean visual acuity in patients with minimally classic or occult choroidal neovascularization related to age-related macular degeneration (ARMD)?[1]

Funding: Genentech and Novartis Pharma.

Year Study Began: 2003.

Year Study Published: 2006.

[*] Basic and Clinical Science Course, Section 12. *Retina and Vitreous*. San Francisco: American Academy of Ophthalmology; 2018–2019: 80–82, 87.

Study Location: 96 sites in the United States.

Who Was Studied: Patients, 50 years of age or older, had primary or recurrent choroidal neovascularization associated with AMD, involving the foveal center, assessed with the use of fluorescein angiography and fundus photography as minimally classic or occult with no classic choroidal neovascularization; the maximum lesion size was 12 optic-disc areas, with neovascularization composing 50% or more of the entire lesion. There had to be evidence of presumed recent progression of disease (observable blood, recent vision loss, or a recent increase in a lesion's greatest linear diameter of 10% or more), and a best corrected visual acuity of 20/40 to 20/320.

Who Was Excluded: Patients were ineligible if they had had prior treatment with verteporfin photodynamic therapy, external-beam radiation therapy, or transpupillary thermotherapy, or intraocular surgery in the study eye, or uncontrolled glaucoma.

How Many Patients: 716.

Study Overview: MARINA was a 2-year, randomized, double-blind, sham-controlled study (Figure 40.1).[1]

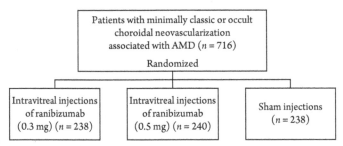

Figure 40.1 Summary of MARINA.

Study Intervention: Patients were randomly assigned to receive monthly intravitreal injections of ranibizumab at a dose of either 0.3 mg or 0.5 mg or sham injections monthly for 2 years in 1 eye.

Follow-Up: 2 years (with a prespecified primary efficacy analysis at 12 months).

Endpoints: The primary endpoint was the proportion of patients losing fewer than 15 letters from baseline visual acuity at 12 months.

RESULTS

- At 12 months, 94.5% of the patients receiving 0.3 mg ranibizumab and 94.6% of those receiving 0.5 mg ranibizumab had lost fewer than 15 letters from baseline visual acuity, as compared with 62.2% in the sham-injection group ($P < .001$ for the comparison of each dose with the sham-injection group).
- Visual acuity improved by 15 or more letters in 24.8% of the 0.3-mg ranibizumab group and 33.8% of the 0.5-mg ranibizumab group, as compared with 5.0% of the sham-injection group ($P < .001$ for both doses).
  - Mean increases in visual acuity were 6.5 letters in the 0.3-mg ranibizumab group and 7.2 letters in the 0.5-mg ranibizumab group, as compared with a decrease of 10.4 letters in the sham-injection group ($P < .001$ for both comparisons).
- At 24 months, 92.0% of the patients receiving 0.3 mg of ranibizumab and 90.0% of those receiving 0.5 mg had lost fewer than 15 letters from baseline visual acuity, as compared with 52.9% in the sham-injection group ($P < .001$ for each comparison).
- At both doses of ranibizumab, the mean improvement from baseline in visual-acuity scores was evident 7 days after the first injection ($P = .006$ for the 0.3-mg dose and $P = .003$ for the 0.5-mg dose), whereas mean visual acuity in the sham-injection group declined steadily over time at each monthly assessment ($P < .001$ for both comparisons).
- The average benefit associated with ranibizumab over that of sham injection was approximately 17 letters in each dose group at 12 months and 20 to 21 letters at 24 months.
- During 24 months, presumed endophthalmitis was identified in five patients (1.0%) and serious uveitis in six patients (1.3%) given ranibizumab.
- The overall incidence of any systemic adverse event, including adverse events previously associated with systemically administered anti-VEGF therapy, such as arterial thromboembolic events and hypertension, was similar among the groups.
  - Cumulative rates of nonocular hemorrhage increased in all groups through the second treatment year, but more so in the ranibizumab groups. By 24 months, nonocular hemorrhage had occurred in 5.5% of patients in the sham-injection group, as compared with 9.2% of those receiving 0.3 mg of ranibizumab and 8.8% of those receiving 0.5 mg of ranibizumab; none of the differences were significant.

Criticisms and Limitations: The study was not powered to detect small differences between groups in the rates of uncommon adverse events. The study was also not powered sufficiently to conclude whether these differences were drug-induced or related to chance alone.

Other Relevant Studies and Information:

- Treatment of neovascular AMD with ranibizumab also improves patient-reported visual functions (near activities, distance activities, and vision-specific dependency subscales of the National Eye Institute Visual Function Questionnaire 25 (NEI VFQ-25) in a meaningful way compared with sham treatments.[2]
- An analysis of clinically relevant subgroups of patients in the MARINA study indicated that ranibizumab treatment was associated with an average increase from baseline VA in all subgroups evaluated, and that ranibizumab treatment was superior to sham treatment across all subgroups.[3]
  - The most important predictors of VA outcomes were, in decreasing order of importance, baseline VA score, CNV lesion size, and age.
- A 2-year, multicenter, randomized, double-blind study of monthly intravitreal injections of ranibizumab (0.3 mg or 0.5 mg) plus sham verteporfin therapy or monthly sham injections plus active verteporfin therapy for predominantly classic neovascular AMD showed that ranibizumab was superior to verteporfin as intravitreal treatment, with low rates of serious ocular adverse events.[4-6]

Summary and Implications: Ranibizumab therapy was associated with clinically and statistically significant benefits with respect to visual acuity and angiographic lesions during 2 years of follow-up in patients with minimally classic or occult lesions with no classic choroidal neovascularization. The efficacy outcomes were achieved with low rate of serious ocular adverse events and with no clear differences in the rate of nonocular adverse events compared to the sham group.

CLINICAL CASE: AN ELDERLY MAN WITH "WET" AMD

Case History
A 78-year-old man presents with complaints of sudden-onset blurring of vision and metamorphopsia in the left eye. He has been followed previously for nonexudative macular degeneration. His vision is 20/25 in the right eye and

20/200 in the left eye. Exam shows a 1 disc area gray-green lesion with punctate subretinal hemorrhage. Optical coherence tomography of the lesion shows an irregular retinal pigment epithelial detachment with subretinal and intraretinal edema. Fluorescein angiography shows early and progressive leakage at the site of the lesion. Based on the results of the MARINA trial which treatment would you choose and will the patient's age have an effect?

A. Observation only.
B. Photodynamic therapy with verteporfin.
C. Intravitreal injection of ranibizumab.
D. Intravitreal injection of triamcinolone.

Suggested Answer
Option C. The MARINA study demonstrated a clear benefit of monthly injections of ranibizumab over observation with sham treatment. The ANCHOR study demonstrated ranibizumab's benefit over verteporfin therapy. Triamcinolone was not studied in either the MARINA or ANCHOR studies.

References

1. Rosenfeld PJ, Brown DM, Heier JS, et al.; MARINA Study Group. Ranibizumab for neovascular age-related macular degeneration. *N Engl J Med.* 2006;355(14):1419–31.
2. Chang TS, Bressler NM, Fine JT, Dolan CM, Ward J, Klesert TR; MARINA Study Group. Improved vision-related function after ranibizumab treatment of neovascular age-related macular degeneration: results of a randomized clinical trial. *Arch Ophthalmol.* 2007;125(11):1460–9.
3. Boyer DS, Antoszyk AN, Awh CC, Bhisitkul RB, Shapiro H, Acharya NR; MARINA Study Group. Subgroup analysis of the MARINA study of ranibizumab in neovascular age-related macular degeneration. *Ophthalmology.* 2007;114(2):246–52.
4. Brown DM, Kaiser PK, Michels M, et al.; ANCHOR Study Group. Ranibizumab versus verteporfin for neovascular age-related macular degeneration. *N Engl J Med.* 2006;355:1432–44.
5. Brown DM, Michels M, Kaiser PK, Heier JS, Sy JP, Ianchulev T; ANCHOR Study Group. Ranibizumab versus verteporfin photodynamic therapy for neovascular age-related macular degeneration: Two-year results of the ANCHOR study. *Ophthalmology.* 2009;116(1):57–65.e5.
6. Kaiser PK, Brown DM, Zhang K, et al. Ranibizumab for predominantly classic neovascular age-related macular degeneration: subgroup analysis of first-year ANCHOR results. *Am J Ophthalmol.* 2007;144(6):850–7.

41

Ranibizumab and Bevacizumab for Neovascular Age-Related Macular Degeneration*

Comparison of Age-Related Macular Degeneration Treatments Trials (CATT)

At 1 year, bevacizumab and ranibizumab had equivalent effects on visual acuity when administered according to the same schedule. Ranibizumab given as needed with monthly evaluation had effects on vision that were equivalent to those of ranibizumab administered monthly.

—CATT Research Group[1]

Research Question: What is the relative efficacy and safety of intravitreal injections of ranibizumab and bevacizumab for the treatment of neovascular age-related macular degeneration (AMD)?[1] Does an as-needed regimen compromise long-term visual acuity as compared to a monthly regimen?[1]

Funding: National Eye Institute, National Institutes of Health.

Year Study Began: 2008.

Year Study Published: 2011.

* Basic and Clinical Science Course, Section 12. *Retina and Vitreous.* San Francisco: American Academy of Ophthalmology; 2018–2019: 83.

Study Location: 44 clinical centers in the United States.

Who Was Studied: Participants were 50 years of age or older. Eligible eyes (1 eye per patient) had active choroidal neovascularization secondary to AMD, no previous treatment, visual acuity between 20/25 and 20/320, and neovascularization, fluid, or hemorrhage under the fovea. Active choroidal neovascularization required the presence of leakage, as seen on fluorescein angiography, and of fluid, as seen on time-domain optical coherence tomography (OCT), located either within or below the retina or below the retinal pigment epithelium.

Who Was Excluded: None stated.

How Many Patients: 1,185.

Study Overview: This was a randomized, single-blind, non-inferiority trial (Figure 41.1.).[1]

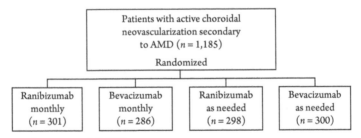

Figure 41.1 Summary of CATT.

Study Intervention: Patients were randomly allocated to 4 groups: ranibizumab every 28 days (monthly), bevacizumab every 28 days, ranibizumab as needed (when signs of active choroidal neovascularization were present), and bevacizumab as needed. Patients receiving the as-needed dosing regimen were evaluated for treatment every 4 weeks and were treated when fluid was present on OCT or when new or persistent hemorrhage, decreased visual acuity relative to the previous visit, or dye leakage or increased lesion size on fluorescein angiography was present.

Follow-Up: 1 year.

Endpoints: The primary outcome was the mean change in visual acuity (VA) at 1 year, with a noninferiority limit of 5 letters on the eye chart.

RESULTS

- Visual acuity improved in all 4 groups between baseline and 1 year, mostly occurring within the first 6 months.
  - Mean change in VA was +8.5 letters in the ranibizumab monthly group, +8.0 in the bevacizumab monthly group, +6.8 letters in the ranibizumab as needed group, and +5.9 letters in the bevacizumab as needed group. Thus, ranibizumab monthly was equivalent to bevacizumab monthly, and bevacizumab as needed was equivalent to ranibizumab as needed. Ranibizumab monthly was equivalent to ranibizumab as needed, but the comparison of bevacizumab monthly and bevacizumab as needed was inconclusive.
  - During the first 36 weeks, the percentage of patients who gained ≥15 letters increased in all 4 study groups and at 1 year there was no significant difference among the groups, ranging from 24.9% in the ranibizumab as needed group to 34.2% in the ranibizumab monthly group.
- The proportion of patients whose visual acuity did not worsen ≥15 or more letters was 94.0% in the bevacizumab monthly group, 94.4% in the ranibizumab monthly group, 91.5% in the bevacizumab as needed group, and 95.4% in the ranibizumab as needed group ($P = .29$).
- The average decrease in thickness of the central retina was greater in the ranibizumab monthly group (196 μm) than in the other groups (152 to 168 μm; $P = .03$).
- Both ranibizumab and bevacizumab dramatically reduced the amount of fluid in and underneath the retina, although the proportion of patients with complete resolution of edema was higher in the ranibizumab groups (27.5% vs. 17.3% at 4 weeks) with the difference persisting throughout the year. The greater prevalence of fluid in the bevacizumab group led to an average of 0.8 more injections per year although the size of the fluid was often minimal.
- Monthly injections of both drugs resulted in no increase in mean lesion size, whereas as needed treatments had slightly larger lesion size.
- No difference was found between the two drugs in death rate, arteriothrombotic events, or venous thrombotic events. However, the rate of hospitalizations was higher in the bevacizumab group (24.1% vs. 19%; $P = .04$). Patients had a higher risk of adverse events if drugs were given as needed compared to monthly.

- The mean number of treatments (up to 13 total) was 7.7 ± 3.5 for the bevacizumab as needed group and 6.9 ± 3.0 for the ranibizumab as needed ($P = .003$).
- For bevacizumab patients, the annual drug cost in this study was $595 in the monthly group and $385 in the as-needed group. For ranibizumab, the annual cost was $23,400 in the monthly group and $13,800 in the as-needed group.

Criticisms and Limitations: Time-domain OCT was used in this study. In clinical practice today, spectral domain OCT is used, which has been shown to be more sensitive in detecting trace fluid warranting treatment compared to time-domain OCT.[2] Time-domain OCT also has lower resolution, so dark areas are often interpreted as edema, which were often not present on spectral domain OCT in one study.[2]

The mean gain of 6.8 letters for ranibizumab as needed and 5.9 letters of bevacizumab as needed is the best result for less than monthly injections compared to previous studies. This was likely explained by changes in treatment parameters. This study specifically set parameters for treatment whenever there was evidence of disease activity (e.g., fluid on OCT) but had no minimal retinal thickness threshold. Previous studies were set according to time or retinal thickness.

It is unknown whether adverse events were related to the drugs themselves or whether it was related to patient's disease state. Cancer patients treated with bevacizumab receive 500 times the dose compared to intravitreal injection without adverse effect. Thus, there is a possibility that some patients are at increased risk of systemic events because of their baseline health status.

Other Relevant Studies and Information:

- In a CATT follow-up study of 1,107 of the original 1,185 patients, in which those initially assigned to monthly treatment were randomly reassigned at 1 year to monthly or as-needed treatment without changing the drug assignment, ranibizumab and bevacizumab had similar effects on visual acuity over a 2-year period.[3]
  - Treatment as needed resulted in less gain in visual acuity, whether instituted at enrollment or after 1 year of monthly treatment.
  - There were no differences between drugs in rates of death or arteriothrombotic events.

- Since the publication of the CATT study, numerous studies in other countries[4-8] and a meta-analysis[9] have confirmed that bevacizumab and ranibizumab for 2 years have equivalent effects on visual acuity.

Summary and Implications: Bevacizumab and ranibizumab had equivalent effects on visual acuity when administered according to the same schedule. Thus, if a patient is unable to afford ranibizumab, bevacizumab could be a useful alternative.

CLINICAL CASE: AN ELDERLY WOMAN WITH NEOVASCULAR AMD

Case History

A 71-year-old white woman presents to the clinic with complaints of decreased visual acuity in her left eye. Her best corrected visual acuity in that eye is found to be 20/40. Examination shows a gray-white lesion in the foveal area with submacular hemorrhage. Optical coherence tomography is notable for presence of intraretinal and subretinal fluid. On fluorescein angiography there is an early hyperfluorescent lesion that increases in size and intensity over time. The patient reports she is uninsured and is asking for the least expensive treatment option. What would you recommend?

A. Intravitreal aflibercept.
B. Intravitreal bevacizumab.
C. Intravitreal dexamethasone implant.
D. Intravitreal ranibizumab.

Suggested Answer

In the CATT study, both ranibizumab and bevacizumab are useful in improving visual acuity in patients with neovascular AMD. The CATT study also evaluated the cost-effectiveness of ranibizumab compared to bevacizumab, and the annual cost was significantly lower in the bevacizumab group. Thus, option B is the best answer.

References

1. CATT Research Group, Martin DF, Maguire MG, Ying GS, Grunwald JE, Fine SL, Jaffe GJ. Ranibizumab and bevacizumab for neovascular age-related macular degeneration. *N Engl J Med*. 2011;364(20):1897–908.

2. Folgar FA, Jaffe GJ, Ying G-S, Maguire MG, Toth CA, the CATT Research Group. Comparison of spectral domain and time domain OCT assessments in the Comparison of Age-Related Macular Degeneration Treatments Trials. *Ophthalmology*. 2014;121(10):1956–65.
3. Comparison of Age-related Macular Degeneration Treatments Trials (CATT) Research Group, Martin DF, Maguire MG, Fine SL, et al. Ranibizumab and bevacizumab for treatment of neovascular age-related macular degeneration: two-year results. *Ophthalmology*. 2012;119(7):1388–98.
4. IVAN Study Investigators, Chakravarthy U, Harding SP, Rogers CA, et al. Ranibizumab versus bevacizumab to treat neovascular age-related macular degeneration: one-year findings from the IVAN randomized trial. *Ophthalmology*. 2012;119(7):1399–411.
5. Chakravarthy U, Harding SP, Rogers CA, et al. A randomised controlled trial to assess the clinical effectiveness and cost-effectiveness of alternative treatments to inhibit VEGF in age-related choroidal neovascularisation (IVAN). *Health Technol Assess*. 2015;19(78):1–298.
6. Kodjikian L, Souied EH, Mimoun G, et al.; GEFAL Study Group. Ranibizumab versus bevacizumab for neovascular age-related macular degeneration: results from the GEFAL noninferiority randomized trial. *Ophthalmology*. 2013;120(11):2300–9.
7. Berg K, Pedersen TR, Sandvik L, Bragadóttir R. Comparison of ranibizumab and bevacizumab for neovascular age-related macular degeneration according to LUCAS treat-and-extend protocol. *Ophthalmology*. 2015;122(1):146–52.
8. Berg K, Hadzalic E, Gjertsen I, et al. Ranibizumab or bevacizumab for neovascular age-related macular degeneration according to the Lucentis Compared to Avastin Study treat-and-extend protocol: two-year results. *Ophthalmology*. 2016;123(1):51–9.
9. Jiang S, Park C, Barner JC. Ranibizumab for age-related macular degeneration: a meta-analysis of dose effects and comparison with no anti-VEGF treatment and bevacizumab. *J Clin Pharm Ther*. 2014;39(3):234–9.

42

Effect of Pre-Enucleation Radiation on Mortality in Large Choroidal Melanomas[*]

The Collaborative Ocular Melanoma Study (COMS) Randomized Trial of Pre-enucleation Radiation of Large Choroidal Melanoma

Initial mortality findings from this clinical trial of pre-enucleation radiation of large choroidal melanoma provide no evidence of a survival difference between enucleation alone and pre-enucleation radiation administered in accord with the COMS fractionation schedule.

—*COMS Report No. 10*[1]

Research Question: Does pre-enucleation external radiation to the globe and orbit significantly prolong a patient's lifespan compared to standard enucleation alone?[1]

Funding: National Eye Institute, National Institutes of Health.

Year Study Began: 1986.

Year Study Published: 1998.

Study Location: 43 clinical centers in the United States and Canada.

---

[*] Basic and Clinical Science Course, Section 4. *Ophthalmic Pathology and Intraocular Tumors.* San Francisco: American Academy of Ophthalmology; 2018–2019: 253, 271–279.

Who Was Studied: Patients 21 years of age or older with unilateral primary choroidal melanoma that was 2.0 mm or greater in apical height and greater than 16.0 mm in longest basal diameter, or greater than 10.0 mm in apical height regardless of the basal dimensions. Patients with peripapillary choroidal melanoma (defined as those with the proximal tumor border closer than 2.0 mm to the optic disc) greater than 8.0 mm in apical height were also eligible. Also, eligible patients had no other primary tumor, no history of cancer (other than noninvasive nonmelanotic skin cancer or carcinoma in situ of the uterine cervix), were judged to be free of metastatic melanoma (by an internist/oncologist), and had a presumed life expectancy greater than 5 years.

Who Was Excluded: Patients were excluded if they had previous treatment for choroidal or ciliary body melanoma in either eye, treatment for any condition secondary to the tumor, or fine-needle aspiration biopsy of the melanoma. Also, patients who had extrascleral tumor extension of 2.0 mm or more visible during echography or clinical exam, who had diffuse, ring, or multifocal tumors, or who had tumors that were judged to be predominantly ciliary body melanoma were ineligible. Use of immunosuppressive therapy was also grounds for ineligibility.

How Many Patients: 1,003.

Study Overview: COMS was a randomized clinical trial (Figure 42.1).[1-3]

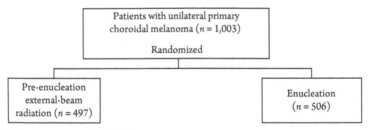

Figure 42.1 Summary of COMS.

Study Intervention: Patients were randomly allocated to enucleation alone or pre-enucleation external-beam radiation. The pre-enucleation radiation group was given 20 Gy of external radiation to the orbit and globe prior to enucleation (generally administered over 5 sessions within an 8-day span); the enucleation group underwent enucleation only.

Follow-Up: 5 years.

Endpoints: The primary outcome was time to death from any cause.

RESULTS

- The estimated 5-year cumulative survival rates were 57% (95% CI, 52–62) for enucleation alone and 62% (95% CI, 57–66) for pre-enucleation radiation ($P = .32$).
  - After adjusting for time since enrollment, the pre-enucleation radiation group had a reduction in mortality (improvement in survival) of 9% compared to the standard enucleation group.
- The estimated median survival time was 82 months in the enucleation alone group and 94 months in the pre-enucleation radiation group (exact estimates were not available when the paper was published).
- Based on review of 435 (95%) of the 457 deaths, more than 60% of all deaths were attributed to metastatic melanoma, based on histologic confirmation.
  - In the enucleation group, 130 (26%) had died of histologically confirmed metastatic melanoma compared to 139 patients (28%) assigned to pre-enucleation radiation.
  - Five-year survival rates for this outcome were 72% (95% CI, 68–76) after enucleation alone and 74% (95% CI, 69–78) after pre-enucleation radiation ($P = .64$, log rank test).
- Among the baseline variable evaluated, only older age and maximum tumor basal diameter affected the prognosis for survival to a statistically significant degree.

Criticism and Limitations: The COMS had strict inclusion and exclusion criteria; however, the characteristics of COMS patients were similar to those reported for patients in nonrandomized evaluations and these results can be considered generalizable to most patients with large choroidal melanomas.

For a substantial number of deceased patients, metastatic melanoma could be neither confirmed nor definitely ruled out as the cause of death, a difficulty reported in other such studies.

Other Relevant Studies and Information:

- The COMS 10-year mortality findings confirmed that there is no survival advantage attributable to pre-enucleation radiation.[4]

- Ten-year rates of death with histopathologically confirmed melanoma metastasis were 45% in the pre-enucleation radiation arm and 40% in the enucleation alone arm.
- In the COMS randomized clinical trial of ^{125}I brachytherapy vs. enucleation for treatment of medium choroidal melanoma, mortality rates following [125] I brachytherapy did not differ from mortality rates following enucleation for up to 12 years after treatment.[5,6]
  - The unadjusted estimated 5-year survival rates were 81% in the enucleation arm and 82% in the brachytherapy arm ($P = .48$, log-rank test).
  - By 12 years, cumulative all-cause mortality was 43% among patients in the ^{125}I brachytherapy arm and 41% among those in the enucleation arm.

Summary and Implications: Pre-enucleation external-beam radiation (20 Gy) to the orbit for large choroidal melanoma does not improve survival compared with enucleation alone. It was found, however, to reduce the risk of orbital recurrence. This study established the appropriateness of primary enucleation alone in managing large choroidal melanomas not amenable to globe-conserving therapy.

CLINICAL CASE: COUNSELING A PATIENT WITH LARGE CHOROIDAL MELANOMA

Case History

A 71-year-old man presents to your clinic for an initial visit from a referring provider due to suspicion of a choroidal melanoma in the right eye. He has a past medical history of high blood pressure. The patient states that his vision has declined in the last 1–2 years in the right eye, but notes that the left eye is doing well. He has no history of cancer, is not immunosuppressed, and has no history of ocular surgery or disease. On examination his visual acuity is counting fingers in the right eye and 20/20 in the left eye. There is no relative afferent pupillary defect. His extraocular movements are full and intraocular pressures are 15 mm Hg in both eyes by tonopen. The anterior segment exam is unremarkable. Dilated exam of the right eye reveals a large and elevated pigmented subretinal mass just temporal to the macula. The mass has adjacent subretinal fluid that extends into the macula and appears to have orange pigment scattered over its surface. B-scan ultrasound shows that the apical height of the lesion is 11 mm. The exam findings, in particular the likelihood of ocular melanoma, are discussed with the patient. How would you counsel this patient regarding his treatment options?

A. Recommend pre-enucleation external beam radiation (20 Gy), since this is a proven way to decrease death from metastasis.
B. Recommend observation.
C. Recommend enucleation alone.
D. Recommend plaque brachytherapy.

Suggested Answer

Option C is the best answer according to the COMS trial, which showed that pre-enucleation radiation with 20 Gy did not improve survival compared with enucleation alone.

References

1. The Collaborative Ocular Melanoma Study (COMS) randomized trial of pre-enucleation radiation of large choroidal melanoma II: initial mortality findings. COMS report no. 10. *Am J Ophthalmol*. 1998;125:779–96.
2. Collaborative Ocular Melanoma Study Group. Design and methods of a clinical trial for a rare condition: the Collaborative Ocular Melanoma Study. COMS report no. 3. *Controlled Clin Trials*. 1993;14:362–91.
3. Collaborative Ocular Melanoma Study Group. The Collaborative Ocular Melanoma Study (COMS) trial of preenucleation radiation of large choroidal melanoma, I: characteristics of patients enrolled and not enrolled. COMS report no. 9. *Am J Ophthalmol*. 1998;125:767–78.
4. Hawkins BS; Collaborative Ocular Melanoma Study Group. The Collaborative Ocular Melanoma Study (COMS) randomized trial of pre-enucleation radiation of large choroidal melanoma: IV. Ten-year mortality findings and prognostic factors. COMS report number 24. *Am J Ophthalmol*. 2004;138(6):936–51.
5. Collaborative Ocular Melanoma Study Group: The COMS randomized trial of iodine 125 brachytherapy for choroidal melanoma. III. Initial mortality findings. COMS Report No. 18. *Arch Ophthalmol*. 119:969–82, 2001.
6. Collaborative Ocular Melanoma Study Group. The COMS randomized trial of iodine 125 brachytherapy for choroidal melanoma: V. Twelve-year mortality rates and prognostic factors: COMS report No. 28. *Arch Ophthalmol*. 2006;124(12):1684–93.

43

Systemic Anti-Inflammatory Therapy Versus Fluocinolone Acetonide*

Multicenter Uveitis Steroid Treatment (MUST) Trial and Follow-Up Study

Based on cost effectiveness and side-effect considerations, systemic therapy may be indicated as the initial treatment for many bilateral uveitis cases. However, implant therapy is a reasonable alternative, especially for unilateral cases and when systemic therapy is not feasible or is not successful.

—MUST TRIAL RESEARCH GROUP[1]

Research Question: Is a surgically placed fluocinolone acetonide intravitreous implant as effective as systemic corticosteroids (supplemented by corticosteroid-sparing immunosuppressive drugs when indicated) for the treatment of intermediate uveitis, posterior uveitis, and panuveitis?[1]

Funding: National Eye Institute, National Institutes of Health; Bausch & Lomb (Rochester, NY); Research to Prevent Blindness (New York, NY); Paul and Evanina Mackall Foundation (New York, NY).

Year Study Began: 2005.

* Basic and Clinical Science Course, Section 9. *Intraocular Inflammation and Uveitis*. San Francisco: American Academy of Ophthalmology, 2018–2019: 98–99.

Year Study Published: 2015.

Study Location: 23 centers in the United States, United Kingdom, and Australia.

Who Was Studied: Participants, 13 years of age or older with active or recently active (within ≤60 days) noninfectious intermediate uveitis, posterior uveitis, or panuveitis in one or both eyes for which systemic corticosteroid therapy was indicated. (Most patients' uveitis was controlled satisfactorily at the time of entry into the MUST Trial Follow-up Study, and they continued their originally assigned treatment.)

Who Was Excluded: Patients requiring systemic therapy for nonocular indications at the time of enrollment and those for whom 1 of the treatments was contraindicated.

How Many Patients: 255.

Study Overview: The Multicenter Uveitis Steroid Treatment (MUST) Trial was a randomized, partially masked, parallel treatment comparative effectiveness trial (Figure 43.1).[1,2]

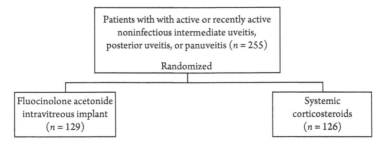

Figure 43.1 Summary of the MUST Trial.

Study Intervention: Patients in the implant arm had initial implantation of a fluocinolone acetonide implant (0.59 mg; Bausch & Lomb, Rochester, NY) after quieting the anterior chamber; the implant was replaced when recurrence of uveitis activity to a level that would justify systemic corticosteroid therapy was observed. Patients in the systemic therapy arm were treated with high doses of systemic corticosteroids sufficient to control active inflammation, followed by tapering and maintenance with as low a dose of corticosteroids as possible, using corticosteroid-sparing immunosuppressive therapy if needed to achieve a suppressive dose that was tolerated and at a level bioequivalent to 7.5 mg prednisone daily or less.

Follow-Up: 54 months.

Endpoints: Best-corrected visual acuity (BCVA); visual field mean deviation (MD); activity of uveitis (anterior chamber cells and vitreous haze), graded by unmasked clinicians using standardized methods; and presence of macular edema on optical coherence tomography (OCT).

RESULTS

- The visual function trajectory in uveitic eyes demonstrated a similar degree of modest improvement from baseline to 54 months in both groups.
  - The mean improvement in BCVA at 54 months was 2.4 and 3.1 letters in the implant and systemic groups, respectively ($P = .73$).
  - Many had excellent initial visual acuity, limiting the potential for improvement. Among uveitic eyes, 50% had a baseline BCVA of 20/40 or better.
- Overall visual field sensitivity as measured by the mean automated perimetry mean deviation (MD) score remained similar to baseline throughout 48 months of follow-up in both groups. However, there was a small excess of cases with lower visual field sensitivity in the implant group, likely corresponding to the higher risk of glaucoma in these patients.
- Overall control of inflammation was superior in the implant group at every time point assessed ($P < .016$), although most eyes in the systemic therapy arm also showed substantial improvement, achieving complete control or low levels of inflammation.
  - Most initially active eyes in both groups were controlled within 9 months of randomization, but significantly more were controlled in the implant group.
  - There was a tendency for systemic therapy-assigned uveitic eyes to have a higher proportion of grade 1+ or greater anterior chamber cells and vitreous haze.
- Although macular edema improved significantly more often with implant treatment within the first 6 months, the systemic group gradually improved over time such that the proportions with macular edema converged in the 2 groups by 36 months and overlapped thereafter ($P = .41$ at 48 months).

Criticisms and Limitations: Losses to follow-up were a problem: by 54 months, 15%–18% of patients were no longer under observation. Crossovers between treatment arms, approximately 20% in each direction, were another problem. This may have diluted differences between treatment arms and resulted in underestimation of the superiority of implant therapy in controlling inflammation, but are unlikely to have affected the primary visual acuity results.

Use of time-domain OCT (rather than the more precise spectral-domain OCT) likely led to a degree of measurement error in both arms of the trial, but is unlikely to have affected assessment of the relative impact of the alternative treatments on macular edema.

Other Relevant Studies and Information:

- The results of an additional follow-up study of the MUST cohort suggested that fluocinolone acetonide implant therapy is associated with a clinically important increased risk of glaucoma and cataract with respect to systemic therapy.[4]
  - Among initially phakic eyes, cataract and cataract surgery occurred significantly more often in the implant group (hazard ratio [HR], 3.0; $P = .0001$; and HR, 3.8; $P < .0001$, respectively). In the implant group, most cataract surgery occurred within the first 2 years.
  - Intraocular pressure elevation measures occurred more frequently in the implant group (HR range, 3.7–5.6; all $P < .0001$), and glaucoma (assessed annually) also occurred more frequently (26.3% vs. 10.2% by 48 months; HR, 3.0; $P = .0002$).
  - Potential complications of systemic therapy, including measures of hypertension, hyperlipidemia, diabetes, bone disease, and hematologic and serum chemistry indicators of immunosuppression toxicity, did not differ between groups through 54 months.
- At 3 years, fluocinolone acetonide implant therapy was reasonably cost-effective compared with systemic therapy for individuals with unilateral intermediate, posterior, or panuveitis but not for those with bilateral disease. These results do not apply to the use of implant therapy when systemic therapy has failed or is contraindicated.[5]

Summary and Implications: Systemic and implant therapies yield similar visual outcomes through 54 months of treatment. Given the greater cost of implant therapy for bilateral disease, and the higher risk of ocular complications in the implant arm, systemic therapy may be the preferred initial therapy for most bilateral cases of active or recently active intermediate uveitis, posterior uveitis, and panuveitis. Implant therapy seems to have a valuable role for severe cases in which systemic therapy has failed, or whenever systemic therapy is not feasible. For unilateral cases, implant therapy seems to be reasonably cost-effective.

CLINICAL CASE: A YOUNG MAN WITH POSTERIOR UVEITIS

Case History

A 23-year-old man with a history of sarcoidosis and diabetes is found to have unilateral posterior uveitis. In your informed consent discussion about implant therapy you refer to the MUST Trial. Which of the following statements is true in regards to outcomes of ocular inflammation and best corrected visual acuity (BCVA)?

A. The MUST trial demonstrated that the degree of ocular inflammation improved faster in the systemic corticosteroid group, although the BCVA showed modest improvement in both groups.
B. The MUST trial demonstrated that control of ocular inflammation was superior in the implant group, although the BCVA showed modest improvement in both groups.
C. The MUST trial demonstrated that the BCVA improved significantly more in the implant group, although the control of inflammation was equal in both groups.
D. The MUST trial demonstrated that the BCVA improved more in the systemic corticosteroid group, although the control of inflammation was equal in both groups.

Suggested Answer

Option B.

References

1. Multicenter Uveitis Steroid Treatment (MUST) Trial Research Group, Kempen JH, Altaweel MM, Drye LT, et al. Benefits of Systemic Anti-inflammatory Therapy versus Fluocinolone Acetonide Intraocular implant for intermediate uveitis, posterior uveitis, and panuveitis: fifty-four-month results of the Multicenter Uveitis Steroid Treatment (MUST) trial and follow-up study. *Ophthalmology*. 2015;122(10):1967–75.
2. Multicenter Uveitis Steroid Treatment Trial Research Group, Kempen JH, Altaweel MM, Holbrook JT, Jabs DA, Sugar EA. The multicenter uveitis steroid treatment trial: rationale, design, and baseline characteristics. *Am J Ophthalmol*. 2010;149(4):550–61.e10.

3. The Multicenter Uveitis Steroid Treatment Trial Research Group, Kempen JH, Altaweel MM, Holbrook JT, et al. Randomized comparison of systemic anti-inflammatory therapy versus fluocinolone acetonide implant for intermediate, posterior, and panuveitis: the multicenter uveitis steroid treatment trial. *Ophthalmology.* 2011;118(10):1916–26.

4. The Multicenter Uveitis Steroid Treatment (MUST) Trial Follow-up Study Research Group. Quality of life and risks associated with systemic anti-inflammatory therapy versus fluocinolone acetonide intraocular implant for intermediate uveitis, posterior uveitis, or panuveitis: fifty-four-month results of the Multicenter Uveitis Steroid Treatment Trial (MUST) and follow-up study. *Ophthalmology.* 2015;122:1976–86.

5. Multicenter Uveitis Steroid Treatment (MUST) Trial Research Group, Sugar EA, Holbrook JT, Kempen JH, et al. Cost-effectiveness of fluocinolone acetonide implant versus systemic therapy for noninfectious intermediate, posterior, and panuveitis. *Ophthalmology.* 2014;121:1855–62.

44

Botulinum A Toxin Injection into Extraocular Muscles as an Alternative to Strabismus Surgery*

> Injection of botulinum A toxin into extraocular muscle to weaken the muscle appears to be a practical adjunct or alternative to surgical correction.
>
> —ALAN B. SCOTT[1]

Research Question: Is injection of botulinum A toxin into the extraocular muscles an effective, safe alternative treatment for strabismus?[1]

Funding: National Institutes of Health and the Smith-Kettlewell Eye Research Foundation.

Year Study Began: Unknown, possibly 1974, based on the botulinum A toxin lot number.

Year Study Published: 1980.

Study Location: Single physician clinic in San Francisco, CA.

---

* Basic and Clinical Science Course, Section 6. *Pediatric Ophthalmology and Strabismus*. San Francisco: American Academy of Ophthalmology; 2018–2019: 175–176.

Who Was Studied: Patients with multiple types of strabismus with different etiologies. Some patients had previously been treated surgically.

Who Was Excluded: Not specified.

How Many Patients: 19.

Study Overview: This was a case series describing the use of botulinum A toxin for the treatment of strabismus.

Study Intervention: Purified botulinum A toxin was injected into the appropriate intraocular muscle at an initial concentration of 6.25×10^{-5} micrograms or 3.12×10^{-4} micrograms. On follow-up, this concentration was either increased or decreased based on the initial response. To ensure the injection was going into the muscle, the needle had an electromyogram tip to record muscle activity while injecting the medication.

Follow-Up: Not specified, and appeared to vary among the patients. Most seemed to get a 2-day follow up and 3-month follow-up. Based on 1 graph in the paper, the patients were seen every 10 days to measure change in strabismus.

Endpoints: An endpoint was not specifically stated, but the effect of the injection into the extraocular muscle was graded at an unknown time point after injection, either as mild (change in primary position up to 10 prism diopters of alignment maintained for 7 days), moderate (change of up to 20 prism diopters for 30 days), marked (change of up to 30 prism diopters for 60 days), or extended (overcorrection that lasted beyond 60 days).

RESULTS

- The maximum time of paralysis occurred 4 to 5 days following the injection, and then gradually diminished, depending on the dose. The maximum correction of strabismus was 40 prism diopters.
- The paralytic effect correlated with the dose of toxin injected—a concentration of 6.25×10^{-5} micrograms produced mild effect, 3.12×10^{-4} micrograms produced moderate effect, 1.56×10^{-3} micrograms produced marked effect, and 7.8×10^{-3} micrograms produced marked effect. At the 6.25×10^{-5} microgram dose, all patients required retreatment, and concentrations less than 6.25×10^{-5} micrograms produced no effect on strabismus.
- No systemic side effects were noted in any patient following injection of botulinum A toxin into the muscle. There was only one case that had

involvement of adjacent extraocular muscles that resolved following day 2, otherwise there were no unwanted ocular side effects documented.

Criticisms and Limitations: This was the first case series describing the use botulinum A toxin for strabismus correction, and it led the way to further studies on the subject, which eventually led to FDA approval in 1990. Since it is a case series it does not have as much validity as a clinical trial would and there is more potential for bias. A prospective trial or even a retrospective review comparing surgical outcomes versus botulinum toxin injection would have made this a stronger study, but for its time it served its purpose. Furthermore, the sample size was small at only 19 patients. The paper itself did not specify standardized follow-up times for the patients. It also did not mention at what time point the initial designation of the effect (mild, moderate, marked, etc.) was made. The sociodemographic characteristics of the patients were not given, and there was no mention of inclusion/exclusion criteria. In fact, some of the patients that were in the series had previously had traditional strabismus surgery. In these patients with previous surgery, it is unknown how stable the strabismus was prior to receiving botulinum A injection.

Other Relevant Studies and Information:

- A Cochran review on the subject included 6 randomized clinical trials published through 2016.[2]
  - Overall, botulinum toxin was found to reduce the angle of deviation by an amount comparable to surgical intervention.
    - Results of botulinum A toxin injection were comparable to surgery in types of strabismus that have potential for binocular vision, including acute onset esotropia, 6th nerve palsy, and infantile esotropia.
    - There was poorer treatment effect with botulinum toxin compared to surgery in patients with horizontal strabismus without potential for binocular vision.
  - The most common adverse effects included ptosis, transient vertical deviation, and intolerable diplopia. Overall, about one-third of patient developed transient ptosis. No systemic side effects were noted in any of the studies.

Summary and Implications: Injection of botulinum A toxin into extraocular muscle to weaken the muscle is a safe and effective alternative (or adjunct) to surgery for strabismus correction. Based on subsequent observational studies and clinical trials since this initial case series, it is important to stratify patients based on the type of strabismus. Current pediatric ophthalmologists use botulinum toxin in acute onset esotropia, 6th nerve palsy, infantile esotropia, or residual strabismus following horizontal muscle surgery.[3]

QUESTION: AN ELDERLY MAN WITH A TRAUMATIC LATERAL RECTUS PALSY

Case History
A 63-year-old man with no significant ocular history but with a significant cardiac history and chronic obstructive pulmonary disease sustains head trauma that results in a traumatic cranial nerve VI palsy on the left side. He has been patching 1 eye to symptomatically relieve his diplopia, but he is tired of patching. On exam you note that the patient has good vision in each eye and the exam is significant for a large esotropia of the left eye. The patient has early cataracts on exam but no other abnormal findings. With his extensive medical history, he is not a good surgical candidate. What would you recommend to the patient as his best treatment option at this time?

A. Atropine drops to the left eye to blur the vision.
B. Neurosurgery evaluation for intracranial options to repair the 6th nerve palsy.
C. Botox injection to the lateral rectus muscle on the left side.
D. Botox injection to the medial rectus muscle on the left side.

Suggested Answer
The correct answer is option D. In this case the lateral rectus muscle in the left eye is not functioning due to the cranial nerve VI palsy, resulting in a left esotopia due to the normal/unopposed action of the medial rectus. Injection of botulinum A toxin into the left medial rectus to weaken the muscle is an alternative to strabismus surgery.

References

1. Scott AB. Botulinum toxin injection into extraocular muscles as an alternative to strabismus surgery. *Ophthalmology*. 1980;87:1044–9.
2. Rowe FJ, Noonan CP. Botulinum toxin for the treatment of strabismus. *Cochrane Database Syst Rev*. 2017;3:CD006499.

3. Gabrielle Weiner interviewing Alejandra de Alba Campomanes, MD, MPH, David G. Hunter, MD, PhD, and Gregg T. Lueder. Reassessing botulinum toxin for childhood strabismus. *EyeNet Magazine*, February 2019 (August 2012). https://www.aao.org/eyenet/article/reassessing-botulinum-toxin-childhood-strabismus. Accessed 2/25/2019.

45

Botulinum A Toxin Injection as a Treatment for Blepharospasm*

Botulinum A toxin injection into the orbicularis oculi muscle is a safe, simple, repeatable, and symptomatically helpful treatment for blepharospasm.

—Scott et al[1]

Research Question: Is injection of botulinum A toxin into the orbicularis oculi muscle a safe and effective treatment for symptomatic relief in patients with essential blepharospasm?

Funding: National Institutes of Health.

Year Study Began: Unknown, possibly 1982.

Year Study Published: 1985.

Study Location: 2 centers in the United States.

Who Was Studied: Patients with a clinical diagnosis of blepharospasm, made on the basis of history of progressive difficulty with eyelid opening and on the clinical finding of bilateral involuntary spasmodic closure of the eyelids. Patients

---

* Basic and Clinical Science Course, Section 7. *Orbit, Eyelids and Lacrimal System*. San Francisco: American Academy of Ophthalmology; 2018–2019: 227–228.

with Meige's syndrome (dystonic movements of other facial muscles) were included. Four patients also had hand apraxia, four had overt cerebrovascular disease, and one had parkinsonism.

Who Was Excluded: 20 patients with follow up of less than 6 months were excluded, as were those with hemifacial spasm and orbicularis myokymia.

How Many Participants: 39.

Study Overview: This was a case series describing the use of botulinum A toxin for the treatment of blepharospasm.

Study Intervention: Botulinum A toxin was injected into the orbicularis oculi muscle and other facial muscles using a 27- or 30-gauge needle, without anesthetic. The dosages, placement, and solution quantity were varied to establish optimal effects. Patients were reinjected when the debilitating symptoms recurred. Preinjection and postinjection video recording of eye blinking and electromyographic monitoring were done in some patients. The isometric force of eyelid closure was measured in most patients before and after injection with a modified calibrated spring-loaded speculum or other force gauge.

Follow-Up: Not specified, and appeared to vary between the patients. Following injection, patients were seen or contacted twice the first week, at weekly intervals for the next 3 weeks, and at monthly intervals thereafter.

Endpoints: Interval between injections (as an indicator of duration of clinical effect); orbicularis muscle force during maximum closure; frequency of side effects (ptosis, strabismus, reported tearing and dryness).

RESULTS

- All of the patients injected with botulinum A toxin into the orbicularis oculi experienced some relief from their symptoms of blepharospasm. The duration of beneficial response varied, increasing with increasing doses of the drug.
  - Patients who were administered doses greater than 20 units per eye were less likely to return within 8 weeks compared with those patients who received smaller doses.

- If the spasm-free interval after injection is less than 3 months, then dosage is increased by 50% on subsequent injections, usually until ptosis begins to occur as a limiting side effect.
- By trial and error, the optimum regimen was found to comprise multiple, subcutaneous injections, using a solution of 5 units/0.1 mL, avoiding the center of the upper lid (to reduce the risk of ptosis and hypotropia) and the central or medial part of the lower lid (to avoid entropion and sagging of the lower lid).
- Transient ptosis was the most common side effect, followed by tearing and dry eye symptoms. Diplopia was a rare reported side effect.
- The treatment was less helpful in patients with marked apraxia of eyelid opening in addition to orbicularis spasm (those with associated hand apraxia, parkinsonism, and Meige's syndrome).

Criticisms and Limitations: This was a case series describing the use of botulinum A toxin for blepharospasm in a relatively small group of patients. While initially 4 patients in the series were injected with saline on one side as a placebo effect, this practice was quickly abandoned since the response difference was so great. However, there was no attempt to make any other comparisons in treatment effect (it would have been insightful if dose and/or injection site comparisons were made between right and left sides in patients in this bilateral disease). It was also noted that patient symptoms returned before full eyelid closure force had returned, which we know to be true. However, no further study was done to attempt to objectify the need for repeat injections other than the patient's symptoms.

Other Relevant Studies and Information:

- Along with those of Frueh et al,[2,3] this was one of the first reports of the use of botulinum A toxin in the treatment of blepharospasm. More recent studies continue to show that botulinum toxin A is an effective, safe, long-term treatment for patients with benign essential blepharospasm and hemifacial spasm.
  - For example, a review of 64 patients treated over more than 10 consecutive years with a mean duration of follow up of 14.1 ± 3.1 years (range 10–20 years) showed that the mean durations of effect during the first and last years of treatment were 12.4 ± 7.1 and 14.6 ± 7.0 weeks, respectively ($P = .076$).

Summary and Implications: Botulinum A toxin injection into the orbicularis oculi muscle is a safe, simple, and symptomatically helpful treatment for blepharospasm that can be repeated at intervals as required.

CLINICAL CASE: A YOUNG WOMAN WITH BLEPHAROSPASM

Case History
A 41-year-old woman presents for evaluation of eyelid symptoms that have been present for several years but continue to worsen. She states that her eyes constantly blink uncontrollably while she is awake, and that bright lights worsen the blinking to the point where she can no longer drive due to the sunlight causing her eyes to close. She is diagnosed with benign essential blepharospasm and is given botulinum injections into the orbicularis muscles on both sides. What is the side effect she is most likely to experience following the injections?

A. Blurring of vision.
B. Headache.
C. Red eyes.
D. Transient ptosis.

Suggested Answer
The correct answer is option D. According to the case series of Scott et al, transient ptosis is the most common side effect following botulinum injection into the orbicularis muscles.

References

1. Scott AB, Kennedy RA, Stubbs HA. Botulinum A toxin injection as a treatment for blepharospasm. *Arch Ophthalmol.* 1985;103(3):347–50.
2. Frueh BR, Felt DP, Wojno TH, Musch DC. Treatment of blepharospasm with botulinum toxin: a preliminary report. *Arch Ophthalmol.* 1984;102(10):1464–8.
3. Frueh BR, Musch DC. Treatment of facial spasm with botulinum toxin: an interim report. *Ophthalmology.* 1986;93(7):917–23.
4. Ababneh OH, Cetinkaya A, Kulwin DR. Long-term efficacy and safety of botulinum toxin A injections to treat blepharospasm and hemifacial spasm. *Clin Exp Ophthalmol.* 2014;42(3):254–61.

46

A Clinical Activity Score That Discriminates Between Inflammatory and Noninflammatory Graves' Ophthalmopathy[*]

The clinical activity score has a high predictive value for the outcome of immunosuppressive treatment in Graves' ophthalmopathy.

—Mourits et al[1]

Research Question: In Graves' ophthalmopathy, is a clinical activity score that differentiates between inflammatory (progressive) and noninflammatory (stationary) disease helpful in patient management?[1]

Funding: None.

Year Study Began: Not stated.

Year Study Published: 1997.

Study Location: The Netherlands.

Who Was Studied: Patients, 20 and 75 years of age, with moderate to severe Graves' ophthalmopathy (defined as having one or more of the following

[*] Basic and Clinical Science Course, Section 7. *Orbit, Eyelids and Lacrimal System.* San Francisco: American Academy of Ophthalmology, 2018–2019: 54–58.

NOSPECS[2] categories: class 2, grade c; class 3, grades abc; class 4, grades abc; and class 6, grade a). All had been euthyroid for at least 3 months.

Who Was Excluded: Patients with diabetes mellitus or with contraindications for corticosteroids or external beam irradiation were not eligible, as were those with rapidly decreasing visual functions or other signs of optic nerve compression by apical crowding. Patients who developed abnormal thyroid function during the study were excluded from the analysis and replaced.

How Many Patients: 43.

Study Overview: This was a retrospective analysis of pooled data from a randomized, double blind, clinical trial comparing oral prednisone and radiotherapy in patients with both inflammatory and noninflammatory Graves' disease.[3] The aim was to determine whether a previously developed index (Clinical Activity Score, CAS)[4] could discriminate between inflammatory and noninflammatory Graves' ophthalmopathy (Figure 46.1).

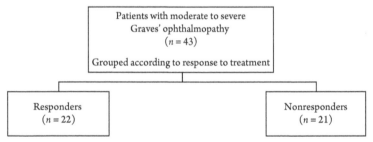

Figure 46.1 Summary of the clinical trial of oral prednisone and radiotherapy for Graves's ophthalmopathy.

Study Intervention: In the original trial patients were randomly assigned to receive oral prednisone and sham irradiation or retrobulbar external beam irradiation and placebo capsules, over 3 months.[3] In this analysis, treatment responders ($n = 22$: 10 in the prednisone group and 12 in the irradiation group) and treatment nonresponders ($n = 21$: 12 in the prednisone group and 9 in the irradiation group) were compared on CAS scores[4] (described below), regardless of treatment allocation.

Follow-Up: None.

Endpoints: The CAS comprises 10 items in 4 categories (Table 46.1).[4] For each item present, 1 point is given; the sum of these points is the CAS, e.g., a CAS of

6 means that 6 items were present, regardless of which items. The CAS was determined in all patients 2 days before treatment started, on the day of the start of treatment, and 24 weeks later by an ophthalmologist blinded to the diagnosis or treatment of the patients. A second ophthalmologist, who was unaware of the CAS scores given, classified patients according to the NOSPECS classification during the same time periods. Success of treatment was defined in an improvement of NOSPECS class. Disease activity was assessed by CAS.

Table 46.1 THE CLINICAL ACTIVITY SCORE

Category	Item No.	
Pain	1	Painful, oppressive feeling on or behind the globe, during the last 4 weeks
	2	Pain on attempted up, side, or down gaze, during the last 4 weeks
Redness	3	Redness of the eyelid(s)
	4	Diffuse redness of the conjunctiva, covering at least one quadrant
Swelling	5	Swelling of the eyelid(s)
	6	Chemosis
	7	Swollen caruncle
	8	Increase of proptosis of ≥2 mm during a period of 1–3 months
Impaired function	9	Decrease of eye movements in any direction $\geq5°$ during a period of 1–3 months
	10	Decrease of visual acuity of ≥1 line(s) on the Snellen chart (using a pinhole) during a period of 1–3 months

RESULTS

- The pretreatment CAS was significantly higher in responders than in nonresponders.
  - The pretreatment CAS was 3.4 ± 2.0 in responders and 2.4 ± 1.2 in nonresponders ($P = .05$).
  - Twelve (55%) of 22 responders and three (14%) of 21 nonresponders had a pretreatment CAS ≥4 ($P < 0.01$).
- Using a pretreatment CAS cut-off point ≥4, the accuracy of CAS in predicting the therapeutic outcome was: specificity 86%, sensitivity 55%, positive predictive value 80%, negative predictive value 64%.
- Patients with a CAS ≥4 had a similar duration of Graves' ophthalmopathy as patients with a CAS <4.

- Twenty-four weeks after the start of treatment, CAS had decreased only in responders (3.4 ± 2.0 to 1.96 ± 1.4; $P < .001$), whereas it did not change in nonresponders (2.4 ± 1.2 to 2.7 ± 1.9; not significant).
- The reproducibility of the total CAS (comparing the score 2 days before treatment started with the score on the day of the start of treatment) was good (kappa = 0.73).

Criticisms and Limitations: The authors reported that the CAS without the last 3 items (which require 2 assessments 1–3 months apart) does not correlate well with response to treatment. Therefore, 2 visits with at least a month in between are required to assess the CAS. However, this is not a major disadvantage as this time can be used to collect data on the patient's status.

Although very specific, the CAS is not very sensitive: 36% of patients with a CAS <4 showed a favorable response to treatment. According to the authors, weighting items on the CAS did not increase the sensitivity. Therefore, the CAS should be used in combination with other parameters of disease activity.

Other Relevant Studies and Information:

- A prospective clinical study comparing the ability of A-mode ultrasonography in combination with the CAS and duration of disease to predict the response to immunosuppression in Graves' ophthalmopathy found that ultrasonography had a good positive predictive value but a poor negative predictive value. By adding the CAS and duration of Graves' ophthalmopathy, the negative predictive value increased considerably. By using this combination, inactive disease could be identified more precisely, permitting rehabilitative surgery at an earlier stage in these patients.[5]
- Newer grading systems include the European Group on Graves' Orbitopathy (EUGOGO)'s severity scales and the VISA Classification (for severity and activity).[6-8]

Summary and Implications: Disease activity (measured by the CAS), and not disease duration, is the prime determinant of therapeutic outcome. The CAS has a high predictive value for the outcome of immunosuppressive treatment in Graves' ophthalmopathy; a high CAS helps to select patients who will benefit from immunosuppressive treatment. A low CAS, however, does not exclude favorable therapeutic results.

CLINICAL CASE: A YOUNG WOMAN WITH GRAVES' OPHTHALMOPATHY

Case History

A 32-year-old woman with Graves' ophthalmopathy attends your clinic. This is the second time you have seen her in 2 months. Her visual acuity, intraocular pressure and dilated fundus exam are all within normal limits. You and the patient note the following signs and symptoms: redness and swelling of the eyelids of both eyes, medial redness and swelling of the conjunctiva of both eyes, and worsening of proptosis >2 mm since her last visit. Using results of the published study "Clinical Activity Score as a Guide in the Management of Patients with Graves' Ophthalmopathy," how do you council this patient regarding her disease and recommended treatment?

A. She most likely has noninflammatory Graves' disease and would therefore benefit from prednisone treatment.
B. She most likely has noninflammatory Graves' disease and would therefore benefit from radiotherapy treatment.
C. She most likely has inflammatory/progressive Graves' disease but does not have enough clinical signs/symptoms to justify treatment at this point.
D. She most likely has inflammatory/ progressive Graves' disease and would probably benefit from treatment with either prednisone or radiotherapy at this point.

Suggested Answer

Since the patient has a high (>4) CAS, she will most likely benefit from immunosuppressive treatment (option D) using either prednisone or radiotherapy.

References

1. Mourits MP, Prummel MF, Wiersinga WM, Koornneef L. Clinical activity score as a guide in the management of patients with Graves' ophthalmopathy. *Clin Endocrinol (Oxf)*. 1997;47(1):9–14.
2. Werner SC. Modification of the classification of the eye changes of Graves' disease: recommendations of the Ad Hoc Committee of the American Thyroid Association. *J Clin Endocrinol Metab*. 1977;44(1):203–4.
3. Prummel MF, Mourits MP, Blank L, Berghout A, Koornneef L, Wiersinga WM. Randomized double-blind trial of prednisone versus radiotherapy in Graves' ophthalmopathy. *Lancet*. 1993;342(8877):949–54.

4. Mourits MP, Koornneef L, Wiersinga WM, Prummel MF, Berghout A, van der Gaag R. Clinical criteria for the assessment of disease activity in Graves' ophthalmopathy: a novel approach. *Br J Ophthalmol*. 1989;73(8):639–44.

5. Gerding MN, Prummel MF, Wiersinga WM. Assessment of disease activity in Graves' ophthalmopathy by orbital ultrasonography and clinical parameters. *Clin Endocrinol (Oxf)*. 2000;52(5):641–6.

6. Dolman PJ. Evaluating Graves' orbitopathy. *Best Pract Res Clin Endocrinol Metab*. 2012;26(3):229–48.

7. Barrio-Barrio J, Sabater AL, Bonet-Farriol E, Velázquez-Villoria Á, Galofré JC. Graves' ophthalmopathy: VISA versus EUGOGO classification, assessment, and management. *J Ophthalmol*. 2015;2015:249125.

8. Dolman PJ. Grading severity and activity in thyroid eye disease. *Ophthalmic Plast Reconstr Surg*. 2018;34(4S Suppl 1):S34–40.

47

Corticosteroids in the Treatment of Acute Optic Neuritis*

The Optic Neuritis Treatment Trial

Intravenous methylprednisolone followed by oral prednisone speeds the recovery of visual loss due to optic neuritis and results in slightly better vision at six months.

—BECK ET AL[1]

Research Question: Does treatment with either oral prednisone or intravenous methylprednisolone speed the recovery of vision and improve visual outcome in acute optic neuritis?[1]

Funding: National Eye Institute, National Institutes of Health.

Year Study Began: 1988.

Year Study Published: 1992.

Study Location: 15 centers in the United States.

Who Was Studied: To be eligible for the study, a patient had to be between the ages of 18 and 46 years, have a history consistent with acute unilateral optic

* Basic and Clinical Science Course, Section 5. *Neuro-Ophthalmology*. San Francisco: American Academy of Ophthalmology, 2018–2019: 115–116, 317–318.

neuritis with visual symptoms lasting 8 days or less, and have evidence of a relative afferent pupillary defect and a visual-field defect in the affected eye on examination.

Who Was Excluded: Patients were excluded if they had previously had optic neuritis in the same eye or had clinical evidence of a systemic disease, other than multiple sclerosis, that might cause optic neuritis. (After randomization, two patients were found to have a compressive optic neuropathy rather than optic neuritis; two other patients who did have optic neuritis were found to have connective-tissue diseases.)

How Many Patients: 457.

Study Overview: The Optic Neuritis Treatment Trial was a randomized, placebo-controlled, clinical trial.[1-3] 151 patients were randomly allocated to receive intravenous methylprednisolone; 156 to receive oral prednisone; and 150 to receive placebo (Figure 47.1).

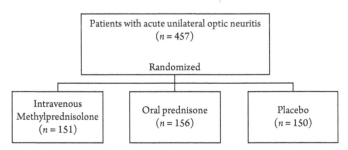

Figure 47.1 Summary of the ONTT.

Study Intervention: The first group was given intravenous methylprednisolone (1 g per day) for 3 days, followed by oral prednisone (1 mg per kilogram per day) for 11 days; the second group received oral prednisone (1 mg per kilogram of body weight per day) for 14 days; the third group was given oral placebo for 14 days.

Follow-Up: 6–24 months.

Endpoints: The primary measures of outcome were visual field and contrast sensitivity; visual acuity and color vision were secondary measures.

Statistical Note: Because of differences between the groups in the degree of visual loss at baseline (a strong predictor of visual outcome), all comparisons of visual function were stratified according to baseline visual acuity.

RESULTS

- The rate of return of vision to normal was higher in the intravenous-methylprednisolone group than in the placebo group (P = .0001 for visual field, P = .02 for contrast sensitivity, and P = .09 for visual acuity)
- At 6 months the distributions for contrast sensitivity (P = .026), visual field (P = .054), and color vision (P = .033) were still significantly better in the intravenous-methylprednisolone group than in the placebo group, although those for visual acuity were not (P = .66)
- Outcomes in the oral-prednisone group did not differ from that in the placebo group.
    - In addition, the rate of new episodes of optic neuritis in either eye was higher in the group receiving oral prednisone than in the placebo group (relative risk for oral prednisone vs. placebo, 1.79; 95%).

Criticisms and Limitations: The patients in the intravenous-methylprednisolone group were not masked as to their treatment assignment; however, it is unlikely that the differences between the intravenous-methylprednisolone group and the placebo group resulted from the lack of masking of the patients, since the personnel examining visual function were usually unaware of the patients' treatment assignments and the differences between groups were evident in several measures of outcome and over the range of follow-up visits.

Although a more rapid rate of recovery was detected in the intravenous methylprednisolone group on day 4—i.e., on completion of the course of methylprednisolone (and in most cases before the initiation of the course of prednisone), it is not possible to say whether treatment with methylprednisolone alone would have been as efficacious as treatment with methylprednisolone and prednisone. It is also not possible to determine whether administering a higher dose of methylprednisolone, or initiating treatment sooner after the onset of symptoms, might have produced even greater benefit than what was found with the dose used in this trial.

The study population was 85% white, so the findings may not apply to populations that have a lower prevalence of optic neuritis (Asian individuals) or different clinical profiles (African American individuals).

Other Relevant Studies and Information:

- Several subsequent (and smaller) studies have similarly reported that the use of intravenous corticosteroids accelerates the recovery of vision but has no long-term visual benefit.[4,5] The most recent (2015) Cochrane Database Systematic Review concluded: "There is no conclusive evidence of benefit in terms of recovery to normal visual acuity, visual field or contrast sensitivity six months after initiation with either intravenous or oral corticosteroids at the doses evaluated in trials included in this review."[6]
- It is widely accepted that oral steroids are contraindicated in patients with acute optic neuritis because their use is associated with a higher recurrence rate—see, for example, the American Academy of Ophthalmology practice recommendations.[7] However, no other study has confirmed the increased recurrence rate of optic neuritis in patients treated with oral corticosteroids.[8]

Summary and Implications: Intravenous methylprednisolone (started within 8 days of symptom onset) followed by oral prednisone speeds the recovery of visual loss due to optic neuritis and results in slightly better vision at 6 months. Oral prednisone alone, as prescribed in this study, is an ineffective treatment and may increase the risk of new episodes of optic neuritis.

CLINICAL CASE: A YOUNG WOMAN WITH ACUTE OPTIC NEURITIS

Case History

A 26-year-old white woman presents to your clinic complaining of blurring of vision in the right eye for the past 3–4 days, associated with seeing flickering lights and feeling a "tugging" sensation behind her eye when she looks in different directions. She has never experienced anything like this before, and denies any history of eye disease or trauma. She suffers occasional unilateral headaches that are associated with light sensitivity. She denies any weakness in extremities but states that sometimes she does notice "tingling" in her left foot. Her only medication is the oral contraceptive pill. She drinks alcohol 2–3 times a week, occasionally "vapes," and denies any illegal drug use.

On examination her visual acuity is counting fingers at 2 feet in the right eye and 20/25 in the left eye. She has a 2+ relative afferent pupillary defect in her right eye. Her extraocular movements are full and she is orthophoric in primary gaze on alternate cover test; however, she does complain of pain with extreme medial and lateral gaze in the right eye. Confrontational visual fields reveal a superior defect in the right eye and are full to finger count in the left eye. Her intraocular pressures are 14 mm Hg in the right eye and 15 mm Hg in the left eye by tonopen. Her color vision is tested—she can't see the plates with the right eye, but gets 11/11 Ishahara plates with the left eye. Her external, lid, and anterior segment exams are unremarkable in both eyes. Dilated fundus exam reveals a hyperemic optic nerve in the right compared to the left with slight blurring of the margins but no obvious elevation. The retina and vasculature are within normal limits in both eyes. What do you recommend to the patient as the best treatment option for her in order to speed up visual recovery in the right eye and decrease risk of recurrence in the near future?

A. Observation only.
B. Oral prednisone 1 mg/kg/day for 14 days.
C. IV methylprednisolone 1 g/day for 3 days followed by oral prednisone 1 mg/kg/day for 10–14 days.
D. IV methylprednisolone 1 g/day for 14 days.

Suggested Answer

The history and examination findings in this patient are typical for acute optic neuritis with marked visual loss in the right eye. Based on the results of the Optic Neuritis Treatment Trial, she should be treated with intravenous methylprednisolone followed by oral prednisone (option C) to speed visual recovery and improve the long-term visual prognosis.

References

1. Beck RW, Cleary PA, Anderson MM Jr, et al. A randomized, controlled trial of corticosteroids in the treatment of acute optic neuritis. The Optic Neuritis Study Group. N Engl J Med. 1992;326(9):581–8.
2. Optic Neuritis Study Group. The clinical profile of optic neuritis: experience of the Optic Neuritis Treatment Trial. Arch Ophthalmol. 1991;109(12):1673–8.
3. Cleary PA, Beck RW, Anderson MM Jr, Kenny DJ, Backlund JY, Gilbert PR. Design, methods, and conduct of the Optic Neuritis Treatment Trial. Control Clin Trials. 1993;14(2):123–42.
4. Kapoor R, Miller DH, Jones SJ, et al. Effects of intravenous methylprednisolone on outcome in MRI-based prognostic subgroups in acute optic neuritis. Neurology. 1998;50(1):230–7.
5. Wakakura M, Mashimo K, Oono S, et al. Multicenter clinical trial for evaluating methylprednisolone pulse treatment of idiopathic optic neuritis in Japan: Optic

Neuritis Treatment Trial Multicenter Cooperative Research Group (ONMRG). *Jpn J Ophthalmol.* 1999;43(2):133–8.

6. Gal RL, Vedula SS, Beck R. Corticosteroids for treating optic neuritis. *Cochrane Database Syst Rev.* 2015;(8):CD001430.

7. American Academy of Ophthalmology Basic and Clinical Science Course (BCSC) 2016–2017. Book 5, Chapter 4 page 119; Chapter 14 page 306.

8. Sellebjerg F, Nielsen HS, Frederiksen JL, Olesen J. A randomized, controlled trial of oral high-dose methylprednisolone in acute optic neuritis. *Neurology.* 1999. 52(7):1479–84.

48

Atropine or Patching for Treatment of Moderate Amblyopia in Children*

Patching vs. Atropine Trial

> Atropine and patching produce improvement of similar magnitude, and both are appropriate modalities for the initial treatment of moderate amblyopia in children aged 3 to less than 7 years.
>
> —THE PEDIATRIC EYE DISEASE INVESTIGATOR GROUP[1]

Research Question: Is treatment with atropine drops as effective as patching for the treatment of moderate amblyopia?[1]

Funding: National Eye Institute, National Institutes of Health.

Year Study Began: 1999.

Year Study Published: 2002.

Study Location: 47 centers in the United States.

Who Was Studied: To be eligible for the study a patient had to be less than 7 years of age, have a visual acuity in the amblyopic eye between 20/40 and 20/100, have a visual acuity in the sound eye of 20/40 or better, have

---

* Basic and Clinical Science Course, Section 6. *Pediatric Ophthalmology and Strabismus.* San Francisco: American Academy of Ophthalmology; 2018–2019: 58–59.

intereye visual acuity difference of 3 or more lines, have an amblyogenic factor meeting study criteria for strabismus or anisometropia, and have had optimal spectacle correction for a minimum of 4 weeks at the time of enrollment into the study.

Who Was Excluded: Patients were excluded if they had any other ocular cause for reduced vision, prior ocular surgery, myopia in either eye, Down syndrome, known skin reaction to patch adhesive, or allergy to atropine drops. After randomization, 1 patient had an amblyopic eye acuity of 20/125, 4 had intereye acuity difference less than 3 lines, and 5 were presumed to have amblyopia but did not have a definite amblyogenic factor.

How Many Patients: 419.

Study Overview: This was a randomized clinical trial (Figure 48.1).[1]

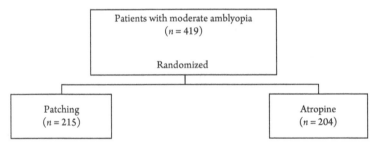

Figure 48.1 Summary of the Patching versus Atropine trial.

Study Intervention: Patients were randomly allocated to patching treatment or to atropine sulfate 1% drops. The patching protocol stipulations included a minimum patching time of 6 hours per day through the total 6 month period. The patching time could be decreased to at least 7 hours per week if criteria for successful treatment were met. The atropine group received 1 drop per day of atropine sulfate 1%, which could be reduced to at least 2 times per week if success criteria were met. If the visual acuity between the 2 eyes became equal, either treatment could be discontinued.

Follow-Up: 6 months.

Endpoints: The primary measure of outcome was visual acuity at 6 months. The primary safety outcome measure was visual acuity in the sound eye. Successful treatment was considered to be acuity of 20/30 or better in the amblyopic eye or improvement of 3 or more lines from baseline. The Amblyopia Treatment Index questionnaire was given to parents at the 5 week interval follow-up.

RESULTS

- At the 5 week interval, visual acuity in the amblyopic eye showed greater improvement with patching than with atropine (2.22-line improvement in the patching group vs. 1.37 in the atropine group—mean difference in logMAR acuity between the groups was 0.087 with a 95% CI of 0.060–0.113).
  - Additionally, at 5 weeks, the percentage of patients that met criteria for successful treatment was higher in the patching vs. atropine group (56% vs. 33%).
- At the 16-week and 6-month intervals, the differences between the group were smaller.
  - At 6 months, the mean change in visual acuity from baseline was 3.16 lines (95% CI, 2.95–3.37) in the patching group and 2.84 lines (95% CI, 2.61–3.07) in the atropine group.
  - At 6 months, the percentage of patients that met criteria for successful treatment was similar between the two groups (79% in patching group vs. 74% in the atropine group).
- At 6 months, only 1 patient in the study (in the atropine group) required treatment for reverse amblyopia in the sound eye, with return to baseline acuity.
- Based on the parent questionnaire given at the 5-week interval, atropine was better tolerated than patching, including better compliance and social stigmata scores.

Criticisms and Limitations: The patients, their parents, and the investigators were not masked to the treatment group assignments. However, this likely had little effect on the outcome of the study, considering that the tester checking visual acuity (the primary outcome of the study) was masked in 97% percent of cases.

The 6-month interval is overall a short-term follow-up for amblyopia. The full benefit of either atropine or patching may be longer than 6 months for some specific patients. Thus, longer a follow-up interval may have shown a higher percentage of patients that would have met criteria for successful treatment.

The study population was also 83% white, so the findings may not apply to populations that have a different clinical profiles.

Other Relevant Studies and Information:

- In 2008 and 2014, 10- and 15-year follow-up data were published, respectively.[2-3] The authors concluded, "At 15 years of age, most children treated for moderate amblyopia when younger than 7 years have good visual acuity, although mild residual amblyopia is common. The outcome is similar regardless of initial treatment with atropine or patching. The results indicate that improvement occurring with amblyopia treatment is maintained until at least 15 years of age."[2]
- Since publishing this study, the Pediatric Eye Disease Investigator group has published data to support patching 2 hours per day (instead of 6 hours) and atropine sulfate 1% given only 2 consecutive days of the week (instead of every day).[4-5] These and other current recommendations for treatment of amblyopia can be found in the American Academy of Ophthalmology amblyopia preferred practice guidelines.

Summary and Implications: Both patching and atropine are equally as effective in the initial treatment of moderate amblyopia. Based on the 5-week data, patching shows faster initial improvement compared to atropine.

CLINICAL CASE: AMBLYOPIA IN A 5-YEAR-OLD BOY

Case History

A 5-year-old boy is brought into clinic by his mother for a routine eye exam prior to starting school. The mother denies any birth trauma or prematurity, and states that his development has been normal up to this point. She says that he appears to see well when he is playing with his toys at home. The patient's father has a history of a "lazy eye."

On examination his visual acuity is 20/100 in the right eye and 20/25 in the left eye. The pupils have normal reactivity without a relative afferent pupillary defect (RAPD). His extraocular movements are full, and he is orthophoric in primary gaze on alternate cover test. Confrontational visual fields are full in both eye. On slit lamp exam, both the anterior and posterior segments of the eye appear normal and healthy. Cycloplegic refraction/retinoscopy reveals a +4.00 sphere in the right and a +1.00 sphere in the left. You prescribe the patient glasses and see him back in 1 month. His visual acuity is now 20/60 in the right and 20/20 in the left. Two months later, the right eye is still 20/60. Based on the patching vs. atropine study, what do you recommend to the patient's parent as the next step in treatment?

A. Continue with glasses only.
B. Continue glasses plus start patching the right eye 6 hours per day.
C. Continue glasses plus start patching the left eye 6 hour per day.
D. Stop glasses completely and start atropine sulfate 1% in the right eye every day.

Suggested Answer

The history and examination findings in this patient suggest amblyopia secondary to anisometropia. The initial treatment of amblyopia includes treating any uncorrected refractive error (as required for any patient entering into the patching vs. atropine study). Based on the study, the sound eye should either be patched (option C) or penalized with atropine drops. Options B and D would penalize the amblyopic eye and make the situation worse.

References

1. The Pediatric Eye Disease Investigator Group. A randomized trial of atropine vs patching for treatment of moderate amblyopia in children. *Arch Ophthalmol.* 2002;120:268–78.
2. The Pediatric Eye Disease Investigator Group. Atropine vs patching for treatment of moderate amblyopia: follow-up at 15 years of age of a randomized clinical trial. *JAMA Ophthalmol.* 2014;132(7):799–805.
3. The Pediatric Eye Disease Investigator Group. Atropine vs patching for treatment of moderate amblyopia: follow-up at age 10 years. *Arch Ophthalmol* 2008;126(8):1039–44.
4. Pediatric Eye Disease Investigator Group. A randomized trial of patching regimens for treatment of moderate amblyopia in children. *Arch Ophthalmol.* 2003:121(5);603–11.
5. Pediatric Eye Disease Investigator Group. A randomized trial of atropine regimens for treatment of moderate amblyopia in children. *Ophthalmology.* 2004:111(11);2076–85.

49

Contact Lens Versus Intraocular Lens Correction of Monocular Aphakia During Infancy*

The Infant Aphakia Treatment Study

> Until longer-term follow-up data are available, caution should be exercised when performing IOL implantation in children aged 6 months or younger given the higher incidence of adverse events and the absence of an improved short-term visual outcome compared with contact lens use.
>
> —LAMBERT ET AL[1]

Research Question: For the correction of aphakia after cataract surgery performed in infants with a unilateral congenital cataract between 1 and 6 months of age, is immediate intraocular lens (IOL) implantation superior to contact lens?[1]

Funding: National Eye Institute, National Institutes of Health and Research to Prevent Blindness.

Year Study Began: 2004.

Year Study Published: 2010.

Study Location: 12 centers in the United States.

* Basic and Clinical Science Course, Section 6. *Pediatric Ophthalmology and Strabismus*. San Francisco: American Academy of Ophthalmology; 2018–2019: 301.

Who Was Studied: To be included in the study patients had to have a visually significant congenital cataract (≥3 mm central opacity) in 1 eye and be between the age of 28 days and 210 days at the time of surgery. If the cataract was due to persistent fetal vasculature, visible stretching of the ciliary processes or involvement of the retina or optic nerve had to be absent.

Who Was Excluded: Patients were excluded if they had acquired cataract, a corneal diameter smaller than 9 mm, a medical condition that might interfere with visual acuity testing, or premature birth (<36 gestational weeks).

How Many Patients: 114.

Study Overview: The Infant Aphakia Treatment Study is a randomized, controlled clinical trial (Figure 49.1).[1,2]

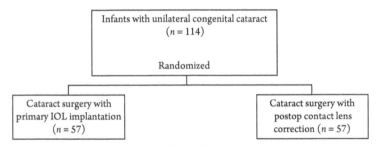

Figure 49.1 Summary of the Infant Aphakia Treatment Study.

Study Intervention: Patients were randomly allocated to have an IOL placed at the time of the initial surgery or to have their eyes left aphakic and corrected with a contact lens. Infants randomized to the contact lens group underwent a lensectomy and anterior vitrectomy. Within a week after cataract surgery, a soft or a rigid gas-permeable contact lens was fitted, with a 2.0-D overcorrection to provide a near-point focus. Infants randomized to the IOL group initially had the lens contents aspirated followed by the implantation of the IOL into the capsular bag (or, failing that, the ciliary sulcus). Following IOL placement, a posterior capsulectomy and an anterior vitrectomy were performed through the pars plana/plicata. Spectacles were prescribed prior to the 1-month postoperative visit or at any later visit, provided that one of the following conditions existed in the treated eye: hyperopia greater than 1.0 D, myopia greater than 3.0 D, or astigmatism greater than 1.5 D. The overall aim was to overcorrect the refractive error by 2.0 D to achieve a near-point focus. In both groups, starting in the 2nd postoperative week, parents were instructed to have their child wear an adhesive occlusive patch over the unoperated eye for 1 hour per day per each month of the child's age until age 8 months. Thereafter, patching was prescribed for all waking hours every other day or for one-half of the patient's waking hours every day.

Follow-Up: 12 months.

Endpoints: The primary measure of outcome was monocular grating visual acuity, tested at 1 year of age by a masked traveling examiner.

RESULTS

- The median logMAR visual acuity was not significantly different between the treated eyes in the 2 groups (contact lens group, 0.80; IOL group, 0.97; $P = .19$).
- More patients in the IOL group underwent 1 or more additional intraocular operations than patients in the contact lens group (63% vs. 12%; $P < .001$).
  - Most of these additional operations were performed to clear lens reproliferation and pupillary membranes from the visual axis.
- There was a trend for a greater occurrence of intraoperative complications in the IOL group (28%) than the contact lens group (11%) ($P = .03$).
  - This was primarily due to a higher incidence of iris prolapse during cataract surgery in the IOL group (21% vs. 4%).
- There was a trend for a higher incidence of strabismus in the contact lens group, but this difference was not statistically significant.
  - At the 12-month examination, 58% of the patients in the IOL group were orthotropic compared with 38% of the patients in the contact lens group ($P = .05$).

Criticisms and Limitations: The proportion of parents in the study reporting excellent adherence in the contact lens group may not be generalizable because the study provided contact lenses, spectacles, and patches at no cost to the patients. Additionally, the regular follow-up interval may have improved compliance. Based on this, it is possible that the study results measure efficacy (benefit under ideal conditions) rather than effectiveness (benefit under normal conditions).

The IOL group was somewhat less adherent to the prescribed patching regimen than the contact lens group, but the differences were relatively small in the first few months after surgery and there was a large amount of variation in patching within both groups.

Other Relevant Studies and Information:

- At 5 years of follow-up, the Infant Aphakia Treatment Study Group reported no significant difference between the median visual acuity of operated eyes in children who underwent primary IOL implantation and those left aphakic. However, there were significantly more adverse events and additional intraoperative procedures in the IOL group.[3]

  - The median logMAR visual acuity was not significantly different between the treated eyes in the 2 treatment groups (both, 0.90; $P = 0.54$).
  - About 50% of treated eyes in both groups had visual acuity less than or equal to 20/200.
  - Significantly more patients in the IOL group had at least 1 adverse event after cataract surgery (contact lens, 56%; IOL, 81%; $P = .02$).
    - The most common adverse events in the IOL group were lens reproliferation into the visual axis, pupillary membranes, and corectopia.
    - Glaucoma/glaucoma suspect occurred in 35% of treated eyes in the contact lens group vs. 28% of eyes in the IOL group ($P = .55$).
    - After the initial cataract surgery, more patients in the IOL group have had at least 1 additional intraocular surgery (contact lens, 21%; IOL, 72%; $P < .001$).

Summary and Implications: There was no statistically significant difference in grating visual acuity at age 1 year between the IOL and contact lens groups; however, additional intraocular operations were performed more frequently in the IOL group. For the treatment of unilateral congenital cataract in in children aged 6 months or younger, the authors recommend leaving the eye aphakic and correcting the aphakia with a contact lens. Given the higher incidence of adverse events and the absence of an improved short-term visual outcome compared with contact lens use, IOL implantation should be reserved for infants who are unable to tolerate contact lenses in order to prevent significant periods of uncorrected aphakia.

CLINICAL CASE: AN INFANT WITH UNILATERAL CONGENITAL CATARACT

Case History
A 4-week-old boy is brought in by his parents who complain of an abnormal red reflex in the infant's right eye that they have noticed in family photos. When looking back through the photos it is apparent that the abnormal

red reflex has been present since birth. Physical exam reveals a dense 4-mm cataract centered in the visual axis. The child had a normal prenatal course and was born by spontaneous vaginal delivery at 39 weeks. No one in the family has a history of congenital cataracts. Further physical examination reveals no other ocular abnormalities of the right eye; exam of the left eye is completely normal. It is determined that the cataract is visually significant. While discussing treatments the mother asks which option will provide the best visual results and best limit the need for further surgery in the future. What is your recommendation?

A. Observation only.
B. Cataract extraction followed by correction with a contact lens.
C. Cataract extraction with primary implantation of an intraocular lens.
D. Spectacles only.

Suggested Answer

Based on the results of the Infant Aphakia Treatment Study (including the 5-year follow-up study), this boy should have cataract extraction followed by correction of aphakia with a contact lens (option B). This approach achieves the same visual outcome as primary IOL implantation, with fewer adverse events and fewer additional surgeries.

References

1. Lambert SR, Buckley EG, Drews-Botsch C, et al.; Infant Aphakia Treatment Study Group. A randomized clinical trial comparing contact lens with intraocular lens correction of monocular aphakia during infancy: grating acuity and adverse events at age 1 year. *Arch Ophthalmol.* 2010;128(7):810–8.
2. The Infant Aphakia Treatment Study Group. The Infant Aphakia Treatment Study: design and clinical measures at enrollment. *Arch Ophthalmol.* 2010;128(1):21–7.
3. Infant Aphakia Treatment Study Group, Lambert SR, Lynn MJ, Hartmann EE, et al. Comparison of contact lens and intraocular lens correction of monocular aphakia during infancy: a randomized clinical trial of HOTV optotype acuity at age 4.5 years and clinical findings at age 5 years. *JAMA Ophthalmol.* 2014;132(6):676–82.

Effect of Acetazolamide on Visual Function in Patients with Idiopathic Intracranial Hypertension and Mild Visual Loss[*]

The Idiopathic Intracranial Hypertension Treatment Trial

In patients with idiopathic intracranial hypertension and mild visual loss, the use of acetazolamide with a low-sodium weight-reduction diet compared with diet alone resulted in modest improvement in visual field function.

—WALL ET AL[1]

Research Question: Is acetazolamide beneficial in improving vision when added to a low-sodium weight reduction diet in patients with idiopathic intracranial hypertension (IIH) and mild visual loss?[1]

Funding: National Eye Institute, National Institutes of Health.

Year Study Began: 2010.

Year Study Published: 2014.

Study Location: 38 academic and private practice sites in North America.

---

[*] Basic and Clinical Science Course, Section 5. *Neuro-Ophthalmology*. San Francisco: American Academy of Ophthalmology; 2018–2019: 110–113.

Who Was Studied: Participants aged 18–60 years were eligible if they met the modified Dandy criteria for IHI (presence of signs and symptoms of increased intracranial pressure; absence of localizing findings on neurologic examination except those known to occur from increased intracranial pressure; absence of deformity, displacement, or obstruction of the ventricular system and otherwise normal neurodiagnostic studies, except for evidence of increased cerebrospinal fluid (CSF) pressure (> 200 mm H2O); abnormal neuroimaging except for empty sella turcica, optic nerve sheath with filled out CSF spaces, and smooth-walled non-flow-related venous sinus stenosis or collapse should lead to another diagnosis; awake and alert patient; no other cause of increased intracranial pressure present) and had reproducible mild visual loss (−2 to −7 dB perimetric mean deviation [PMD]), bilateral papilledema, an elevated CSF opening pressure, and no secondary cause of increased intracranial pressure.

Who Was Excluded: Patients were excluded if there had been total treatment of IIH of more than 2 weeks (except for acetazolamide, limited to 1 week), previous surgery for IIH, previous gastric bypass surgery, abnormal CSF contents, other disorders causing visual loss, optic disc drusen on exam or in previous history, presence of diagnosed untreated obstructive sleep apnea, exposure to a drug, substance, or disorder that has been associated with elevation of intracranial pressure within 2 months of diagnosis such as lithium, vitamin A, or various cyclines, or any other condition requiring diuretics, steroids or other pressure lowering agents including topiramate, or pregnancy.

How Many Patients: 165.

Study Overview: The Idiopathic Intracranial Hypertension Treatment Trial was a randomized, double-masked, placebo-controlled trial (Figure 50.1).[1,2]

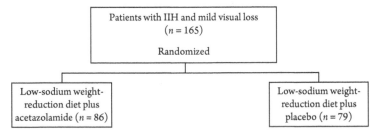

Figure 50.1 Summary of the IIHTT.

Study Intervention: 86 patients were randomly allocated to receive the maximally tolerated dosage of acetazolamide (up to 4 g/day) and 79 were randomly allocated to receive placebo. Both groups were offered a specific dietary plan (a low-sodium weight-reduction diet) and lifestyle modification program.

Follow-Up: 6 months.

Endpoints: The primary outcome was the change in PMD from baseline to month 6 in the most affected eye, as measured by Humphrey Field Analyzer. (PMD is a measure of global visual field loss [mean deviation from age-corrected normal values], with a range of 2 to −32 dB; larger negative values indicate greater vision loss). Secondary outcomes included changes in papilledema grade, visual acuity, quality of life, headache disability, and weight at month 6.

RESULTS

- The mean improvement in PMD was greater with acetazolamide than with placebo (the average difference was 0.71 dB; $P = .050$).
  - Mean improvement in the acetazolamide group was 1.43 dB, from −3.53dB at baseline to −2.10 dB at month 6.
  - Mean improvement in the placebo group was 0.71 dB, from −3.53 dB to −2.82dB at month 6.
- The mean improvement in papilledema grade was greater with acetazolamide than with placebo (the average difference was −0.70; $P < .001$).
  - Mean improvement in the acetazolamide group was −1.31, from 2.76 to 1.45.
  - Mean improvement in the placebo group was −0.61, from 2.76 to 2.15.
- The mean improvement in PMD was greater in participants with a baseline papilledema grade of 3–5 (2.27 dB) than in those with a baseline papilledema grade of 1–2 (−0.67 dB).
- Participants in the acetazolamide group also experienced significant improvement in quality-of-life measures.
- No significant treatment effects were noted with respect to headache disability or visual acuity.
- Participants receiving acetazolamide lost more weight (7.5 kg) during 6 months than those receiving placebo (3.45 kg).
- There were few unexpected adverse events associated with acetazolamide use, and no permanent morbidity.

Criticisms and Limitations: There was a 19% withdrawal rate, although the frequency of, and reasons for, withdrawal were similar in the 2 treatment groups.

The estimated treatment effect on PMD was small (0.71 dB), approximately half of the prespecified minimal clinically important difference of 1.3 dB, which makes interpretation difficult.

Other Relevant Studies and Information: Further analysis of visual field changes over the 6-month study period showed that the acetazolamide group had a significant pointwise improvement in visual field function, particularly in the nasal and pericecal areas; the latter is likely due to reduction in blind spot size related to improvement in papilledema.[3]

- Some participants were categorized as performance failures—they had difficulty in performing the perimetric test, resulting in a marked deterioration in their PMD, but were otherwise stable on repeat examination. Performance failures were found in 21% of subjects and in 2.7% of the total number of visual field examinations and was reversible on repeat testing.[4]
- Seven participants (6 on diet plus placebo) met criteria for treatment failure (defined when the participant's mean PMD worsened ≥2 to 3 dB from the average baseline PMD (range of -2 to -7 dB) with a second retest confirming the visual deterioration). Male patients, those with high-grade papilledema, and those with decreased visual acuity at baseline were more likely to experience treatment failure.[5]

Summary and Implications: In patients with IIH and mild visual loss (defined as having a PMD from −2 to −7 dB), the use of acetazolamide with a low-sodium weight reduction diet resulted in modest improvement in visual field function. The clinical importance of this improvement remains to be determined.

CLINICAL CASE: A YOUNG WOMAN WITH HEADACHES

Case History

A 29-year-old obese Caucasian woman presents to your clinic with a chief complaint of headaches. She has already undergone MRI and MRV imaging and has a report that indicates both of these test were normal with the exception of an "empty sella." She has also had a lumbar puncture, which indicated an opening pressure of 33 cm H_2O but with otherwise normal CSF studies. On your ophthalmic examination, you find that the patient has a Snellen visual acuity of 20/20 in each eye. She has no relative afferent pupillary defect. Her intraocular pressure is 15 mm Hg in each eye. Her anterior segment exam is normal. On dilated fundus exam she is found to have Grade 3 papilledema in each eye. She completes reliable Humphrey Visual 24-2 testing and is found to have −5 dB PMD in each eye. Based on the Idiopathic Intracranial Hypertension Treatment Trial, which statement regarding treatment with both acetazolamide and low-sodium weight reduction diet is true?

A. She is likely to have improvement in PMD, papilledema, and headaches, but unlikely to lose more weight compared with placebo plus diet.
B. She is likely to have improvement in PMD, papilledema, and headaches, but not likely to have improvement in quality of life testing scores as compared with placebo plus diet.
C. She is likely to have improvement in papilledema, headaches, and weight loss, but unlikely to have improvement in PMD and weight loss as compared with placebo plus diet.
D. She is likely to have improvement in PMD, papilledema, weight loss, and have improved quality of life testing scores, but unlikely to have improvement in headache symptoms as compared with placebo plus diet.

Suggested Answer
Option D is the best answer according to the findings of the Idiopathic Intracranial Hypertension Treatment Trial.

References

1. NORDIC Idiopathic Intracranial Hypertension Study Group Writing Committee, Wall M, McDermott MP, Kieburtz KD, et al. Effect of acetazolamide on visual function in patients with idiopathic intracranial hypertension and mild visual loss: the idiopathic intracranial hypertension treatment trial. *JAMA*. 2014;311(16):1641–51.
2. Friedman DI, McDermott MP, Kieburtz K, et al.; NORDIC IIHTT Study Group. The idiopathic intracranial hypertension treatment trial: design considerations and methods. *J Neuroophthalmol*. 2014;34(2):107–17.
3. Wall M, Johnson CA, Cello KE, Zamba KD, McDermott MP, Keltner JL; NORDIC Idiopathic Intracranial Hypertension Study Group. Visual Field Outcomes for the Idiopathic Intracranial Hypertension Treatment Trial (IIHTT). *Invest Ophthalmol Vis Sci*. 2016;57(3):805–12.

4. Cello KE, Keltner JL, Johnson CA, Wall M; NORDIC Idiopathic Intracranial Hypertension Study Group. Factors affecting visual field outcomes in the Idiopathic Intracranial Hypertension Treatment Trial. *J Neuroophthalmol.* 2016;36(1):6–12.

5. Wall M, Falardeau J, Fletcher WA, et al.; NORDIC Idiopathic Intracranial Hypertension Study Group. Risk factors for poor visual outcome in patients with idiopathic intracranial hypertension. *Neurology.* 2015 1;85(9):799–805.

INDEX

Tables and figures are indicated by *t* and *f* following the page number

ABC. *See* Ahmed Baerveldt
    Comparison Study
ABO blood group matching, 1–6
acetazolamide, effect on patients with IIH
    and mild visual loss, 303–307
    clinical case, 306–307
    criticisms and limitations of study, 306
    overview of study, 303–305, 304*f*
    results of study, 305
acrylic intraocular lens (IOL) material,
    53, 54*t*, 56
acute optic neuritis, corticosteroids for,
    285–289
    clinical case, 288–289
    criticisms and limitations of study, 287
    implications of study, 288
    overview of study, 285–287, 286*f*, 287
acyclovir, 12–13
Advanced Glaucoma Intervention Study
    (AGIS), 73–77
    clinical case, 77
    criticisms and limitations of, 76
    implications of, 77
    overview of, 73–74, 75*t*
    results of, 75–76
aflibercept
    for CRVO, 124
    for macular edema after BRVO,
        124, 130

Age-Related Eye Disease Study (AREDS)
    high-dose supplementation for age-related
        cataract and vision loss, 39–44, 41*f*
    high-dose supplementation for AMD
        and vision loss, 219–224, 221*f*
age-related lens opacities. *See* cataract
age-related macular degeneration (AMD/
    ARMD)
    age-related lens opacities, 28
    high-dose supplementation for, 39–44,
        41*f*, 219–224, 221*f*
    neovascular
        bevacizumab for, 251–255, 252*f*
        pegaptanib for, 239–244, 241*f*
        ranibizumab for, 245–249, 246*f*,
            251–255, 252*f*
    photodynamic therapy of subfoveal
        CVN in, 231–236, 232*f*
    prevalence of, 213–216
AGIS. *See* Advanced Glaucoma
    Intervention Study
AGV. *See* Ahmed glaucoma valve
Ahmed Baerveldt Comparison (ABC)
    Study, 109–114
    clinical case, 113–114
    criticisms and limitations of, 112
    implications of, 113
    overview of, 109–110
    results of, 111